What we loved about
The Great Sex Weekend:
Testimonials from experts and "road testers"

"[A] sexy 48-hour getaway guide designed for lovers hoping to rediscover the magic of each other all over again."

—*The Sunday New York Post*

"How long has it been since you and your partner showered together, made love in a new position or lingered in bed all morning? If you can't recall, check out *The Great Sex Weekend*."

—*Glamour*

"What a delicious idea. Rip the list of weekend chores off the refrigerator. Let the grass go unmowed. Throw this book into your overnight bag, along with some of the recommended toys, and go. *The Great Sex Weekend* reclaims time, creating a field of dreams for lovers. Take the *Weekend,* and your love life will benefit for years to come. Become a weekend warrior—for love."

—JAMES R. PETERSON, *Playboy*

This book is like battery cables. Everyone should have it handy to jump start their love life!

"A cornucopia of fun-filled yet practical ways to revitalize and add passion to any sexual relationship."

—LONNIE BARBACH, PH.D., author of
Turn Ons: Pleasing Yourself While You Please Your Lover

After two kids and ten years of marriage, we'd slipped into a sexual rut. The book gave us an incentive to break our pattern. Now we're closer and more open to fun in bed than before.

"The authors . . . cover everything in terms of preparing for the lollapalooza getaway, from how to really make romantic moves to suggesting cozy lodgings in a handful of major cities."

—*New York Newsday*

The Great Sex Weekend forced us to pay attention to each other, which is something we were both hungry for, and didn't even know.

"Helps rekindle the sparks."

—*American Woman*

W9-BJO-996

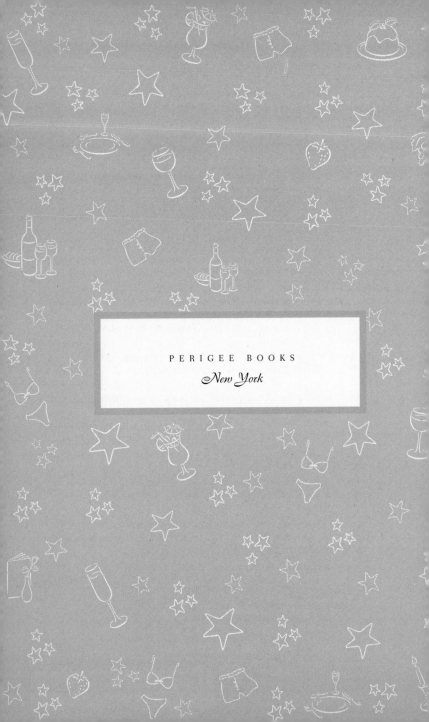

PERIGEE BOOKS

New York

The Great Sex Weekend

A 48-HOUR GUIDE TO REKINDLING SPARKS FOR BOLD, BUSY,* OR BORED LOVERS

Includes a 24-Hour Plan for the Really Busy

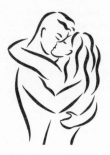

PEPPER SCHWARTZ, PH.D.
and JANET LEVER, PH.D.

A Perigee Book
Published by The Berkley Publishing Group
A division of Penguin Putnam Inc.
375 Hudson Street
New York, New York 10014

Copyright © 1997 by Pepper Schwartz, Ph.D., and Janet Lever, Ph.D.
Book design by Amanda Dewey
Interior illustrations by Paula Munck
Cover design and art by Honi Werner

Photograph of Pepper Schwartz on p. 212 (left) by The University of Washington
Photograph of Janet Lever on p. 212 (right) by Stan Carstensen,
California State University, L.A.

G. P. Putnam's Sons hardcover edition: January 1998
Perigee edition: January 2000
Perigee ISBN: 0-399-52571-8

Published simultaneously in Canada.

The Penguin Putnam Inc. World Wide Web site address is
http://www.penguinputnam.com

The Library of Congress has catalogued the
G. P. Putnam's Sons edition as follows:

Schwartz, Pepper.
The great sex weekend: a 48-hour guide to rekindle sparks for
bold, busy, or bored lovers: includes a 24-hour plan for the
really busy/Pepper Schwartz and Janet Lever.
p.   cm.
ISBN 0-399-14377-7
1. Sex in marriage. 2. Sex instruction. 3. Married people—Sexual
behavior. 4. Married people—Travel. 5. Couples—Sexual
behavior. 6. Couples—Travel. I. Lever, Janet. II. Title.
HQ734.S4155   1998
646.7'8—dc21   97-24094 CIP

Printed in the United States of America

10 9 8 7 6 5 4 3 2 1

To our Road-testers,
for helping us create the weekend,
and to our Partners, who helped us live it

ACKNOWLEDGMENTS

THIS BOOK WAS CREATED WITH THE HELP OF many people. First, we want to thank our agent, Elizabeth Ziemska, for giving us the initial idea; without you, Liz, this book absolutely would not have been written. We also want to thank everyone at Perigee Books, especially Suzanne Bober and John Duff, the editors who gave our drafts the close attention that no one expects these days. And we thank Fran Rosen, too, for her excellent editorial contributions. Rick Kaiser worked long, hard hours getting the manuscript in shape and pursuing countless research leads. Lissa Hall also provided important research assistance.

For their title suggestions, we thank Sandy Berry, River Malcolm, Renee Williams, Gail Zellman, Melissa Trikilis, and Frank Keshishian. Many people gave us advice that made a difference—so many, we fear we may forget a few and apologize to anyone slighted. We thank Peter Adler, Ph.D., Patti Adler, Ph.D., Julie Brown, Angela Cohen, Debra D'Amato, Tom Darden, Ken Dorfman, Sean Dunn, Scott Grusky, Debra Haffner, Lawrence K. Hong, Ph.D., Antoinette T. Hubenette, M.D., Marsha Hunt, O. Lechuga, Holly Lindsey, Monica Mendoza, Stewart Middler, M.D., Mike Neal, Barbara Nellis, Janelle Paige, Skip Paige, Brett Patton, Jennifer Powell, Candida Royalle, Joyce Santo-Diamond, Dean David L. Soltz, Robert Standen, Duane Tudahl, Monique Tudahl, Sandra Wade-Grusky, Ellen J. Wallach, and Milt Williams. And we thank the manufacturers of Albolene and Astroglide, Rebecca Suzanne of Good Vibrations, and Mark Juarez of Tender Loving Things for allowing us to give samples of their products to our road-testers. Thanks to *Philadelphia*, *Washingtonian*, *Seattle*, and *New England* magazines for some of our getaway ideas. We also thank illustrator Malcolm Barter and his publisher, Prometheus, for allowing us to use his drawings from *The Complete Guide to Sexual Fulfillment* as inspiration for some of the illustrations that appear in this book.

Of course, every project is enabled by good friends and family going the distance. Jonathon and Nancy Goodson and Hugh Blake did us a great favor by giving us their lovely beach hideaways in which to write, and Cynthia

Cobaugh helped to proofread and critiqued successive drafts. Janet thanks PJ and Ed Hollister and Sophia and Harry Lever for respecting the priority of this project during a difficult family time. Pepper thanks Cooper and Ryder Schwartz-Skolnik, and especially Art Skolnik, for their constant support and affection and for enduring the many absences that writing this book demanded. Such sacrifices are required by families of all authors, but the irony is greater for a book entitled *The Great Sex Weekend!* (Art, we hope that the promise of future sex getaways—and our thanks—will make up for these lost times.) Finally, we thank all of our road-testers—most of whom chose to remain anonymous—for taking the challenge and sharing details of their intimate experiences. It was their feedback and advice that made it possible for us to refine this program and make it as fun and rewarding as we hope it is.

CONTENTS

Why Most Couples Need This Book

*(And How to Persuade a Reluctant
Partner to Get with the Program)*

Are You Bold, Busy, or Bored?

This book can jump-start your sex life in a single weekend. And if you're like 90 percent of couples who have been together a year or longer, you probably need this program. After the initial days and nights of your relationship when you couldn't keep your hands off each other, everyday life takes over. It is a documented fact: For the majority of couples, even after a short period of time, the frequency of lovemaking decreases dramatically. If you're in the lucky

10 percent who are as sexually active or passionate as you ever were, this book can help you sustain your fabulous sex life. But most couples are not bold sexual adventurers who never miss an opportunity to try something new. More typically, one of the following two scenarios probably sounds familiar to you:

> You and your partner are working hard and have a busy social calendar. You can't believe it, but when you think about it, it's been two weeks since you made love. You think your sex life is important, so you make a mental note that you're going to make love, for sure, sometime this weekend. Friday night you stay out late at a party. By the time you come home, you're both too tired to initiate sex. Saturday is full of errands and you have company coming for dinner on Saturday night. By the time your guests leave, you fall into bed, exhausted. Sunday morning you sleep in. When you finally get up, you do household repairs or job-related work that you can't put off any longer. By late Sunday night, you realize the weekend has slipped by and you didn't make love again.

or

> You and your partner are lying in bed watching television Saturday night. You haven't made love in a couple of weeks and think you really should. You're not really turned on, but you want to be a good part-

ner, so you start stroking your partner's arm. Your partner responds in the same spirit. After a little bit of kissing, you have sex in the predictable, pleasant, but not wholly passionate way that has become part of your intimate life together.

Why don't people have more frequent and inventive sex? In short, they are either busy or bored—or both. Busy people may literally have to schedule sex, but sometimes they don't schedule it often enough, or worse yet, they break their own appointments. A couple's sex life suffers not because they don't love each other or know basic sexual techniques, but because sex always gets put on the back burner. The fast pace of everyday life, especially for people with children, makes it hard for even the most loving couples to have the kind of sex they'd like to have. If couples work different shifts or work weekends and/or nights—or just have an intense life—many weeks can go by before they can find time to make love.

Of course, being busy isn't the only reason for a neglected sex life. Long-term sexual relationships become routine. Each partner knows the other's body so well that they could find each other in a pitch-black room full of a hundred other naked bodies. Over the years, couples get into the habit of making love in exactly the same way. The sex can be satisfying, but often is boring. We all need innovation or surprise—and some permission to experiment—to keep things exciting.

If you think you're good at the basics of sex, but your sexual repertoire isn't as varied as you'd like, rest assured that you are like most Americans. Studies suggest that the range of adult sex play is fairly limited. One national survey found, for example, that just over a third of all couples have taken a shower together and only one in five have bought erotic underwear. Data from a study conducted at the University of Chicago show that even though the vast majority of Americans have experienced oral sex, it is only occasionally included during lovemaking. The same study showed, however, that many Americans find a wide range of sexual activities appealing, even if they haven't found a way to move them from fantasy into their real sex life.

How This Book Can Help You

This book will help you revitalize your sexual and romantic life. We're not just recommending sex in new positions or new places at strange times. Even bold lovers can experience exciting sexual moments that, nevertheless, fail to create intimacy. Building a better sexual partnership requires expanding the emotional connection as well as sexual technique. Our book provides everything couples need for a fast weekend tune-up that really improves their sexual relationship.

This program will help you to create an easy, fun weekend project if you and your partner still have good feelings toward each other but have slipped into bad habits. The Great Sex Weekend provides an occasion to take a short time-out from everyday life and lavish attention on each other. Give us just a few days and we'll help you recapture the desire and playfulness that characterized the early days when you first fell in love.

Just as your car needs to be tuned periodically, every relationship needs to be recharged now and then. Your relationship needs tune-ups that not only keep it going but keep it humming. Think of our play-by-play guide as a handy manual to use again and again to maintain a higher level of sexual desire and satisfaction. When things drift back to where they were before you first tried this program, you'll know what to do. We present more options than you can fit into a single weekend, so there are plenty of ideas and variations for future weekend refreshers.

We expect that you'll return to this book and plan more sexy getaways, because they are fun, and because you are ready to try new ideas. Since readers have different comfort levels with sexual experimentation, we present options ranging from basic to intermediate to exotic. We encourage couples to discuss which ideas are appealing, which might be appealing sometime in the future, and which ideas make one or both partners feel uncomfortable. *Nothing is mandatory.* Every individual's comfort zone differs and must be respected at all times. A few parts of the program are highly recommended because they provide the basic foundation for a creative sex life, but most parts are optional. We invite you to customize the program to your own tastes, but don't be surprised if some of our more exotic suggestions look more enticing the next time you plan a "Great Sex Weekend."

This book is not meant for people with serious sexual

problems. Although our program can be helpful for remo-tivating a partner with low sexual desire, couples whose sexual problems seem bigger than that should seek a good sex therapist. If you need help finding a therapist, ask your doctor or your local family-planning clinic for a referral. You also can send a legal-size self-addressed stamped en-velope to the American Association of Sex Educators, Counselors and Therapists, P.O. Box 238, Mount Vernon, Iowa 52314, and request a list of the nationally certified sex therapists and counselors in your state.

If you're in a troubled relationship, we suggest you wait until things are better before you attempt the weekend program. Couples who are trying to sort out serious prob-lems don't need the extra pressure. The exercises we suggest require goodwill and trust. If the idea of this week-end makes either partner anxious, put it off until it feels right.

How to Get a Reluctant Partner to Cooperate

What if only one partner in the couple thinks the sexual relationship needs to be a few degrees hotter, or if only one of you thinks it's possible to take this much time off to tinker with your sex life? *If your partner is a workaholic and likes the idea but hesitates to schedule a time, suggest the shorter program outlined in "A 24-Hour Plan" at the back of this book.* Plan a date far enough in advance that it is al-most impossible for your partner to refuse. If your partner

claims not to be able to give up even a single day, it's justi-
fiable to say that your relationship not only deserves this
time but that you really want it. When your partner mini-
mizes *the need* for this program, your task becomes more
challenging. Here are a few ideas for convincing a reluctant partner:

1. *Give this book to your partner as a gift that holds the
promise of intimacy and pleasure.* You might even present it
with a bottle of wine and an upbeat card that gives a
choice of three dates. Treat the idea in a lighthearted
manner instead of gravely announcing, "We've got to do
something about our sex life!" Offer the program as a
romp. If it doesn't live up to its full promise, at a minimum
you'll have a great weekend together.

2. *Promote the idea of a sexy getaway as an adventure—something that will require a little reach for both of
you.* Think of a weekend spent improving your sex life as
you might think of taking weekend classes to become a
better cook, photographer, or golfer. Taking lessons does-
n't mean you lack skills; it means you want to be even better at something you really enjoy.

3. *If your partner is good-natured but lazy, offer to take
care of planning the entire weekend.* Book an overnight trip
to a mystery location. All he or she has to do is show up.
Ideally, the planning should be divided so that each partic-
ipant makes it happen. The joint effort creates good feeling right from the start. But it doesn't have to be that way.

If you have a partner who will only participate in this weekend if you make the arrangements, do it as a gift to the relationship. Once you pull it off, your partner may be more inclined to help make the next one happen. Keep in mind, however, that this option works only if you can do all the planning without feeling resentful.

One final word on this topic: Be cautious when presenting the idea of a sexy getaway. You may know you're bored. Your partner may be bored. Your partner may suspect that you're bored. But admitting you're bored might seem hostile. Stick to positive reasons for why you want to take a weekend away together. Point out how your relationship will be strengthened by devoting special time to each other.

Don't pressure your partner—introduce the idea and give him or her time to ponder it. Your partner will probably get over any initial resistance and eventually become intrigued with the idea.

But do persevere. If you don't take this kind of time to nurture your sexual relationship, there's a big price to pay. Besides losing the excitement that good sex provides, over time couples can experience erosion of intimacy and confidence in their personal desirability. With a little time and less effort than you think, you can fix or avoid these problems.

Why This Program Works

The program on which you are about to embark has been tested and works. It was tried on dozens of willing volunteers whom we call our "road-test couples." These included married and cohabiting couples, ranging in age from their twenties to their fifties. Most are heterosexual; a few are same-sex couples. This program worked for both. After following the weekend program, each couple filled out an extensive questionnaire with comments and criticism. Some of their suggestions improved on our original ideas. We quote some of their commentary and tips throughout the book so you can read how other people experienced the weekend program.

We are both professors of sociology who have studied sexuality and intimate relationships for nearly thirty years. Pepper Schwartz is a past president of the Society for the Scientific Study of Sexuality. Both of us teach university courses in human sexuality. And we have worked on major surveys probing people's most private sexual behaviors and attitudes. The results from one study—based on in-depth interviews and questionnaires from 12,000 people—were published in Pepper's book (with Philip Blumstein), *American Couples*. Janet was the senior analyst of the 1982 *Playboy* Readers' Sex Survey, which yielded more than 100,000 responses, making it the largest sex survey ever tabulated.

We publish in popular media as well as academic journals. For the past seven years, we have cowritten *Glamour* magazine's "Sex and Health" column. In addition to answering readers' questions, every month we ask questions of our readers. Their thousands of letters have helped us understand what people want to know and what has helped some of them create an exciting sex life.

In the course of our professional careers, we have used the work of academicians and clinicians in many disciplines. We have picked from the best social science studies, therapeutic models, and other experts' advice to formulate this program. We've put into this book a lifetime of knowledge and interest in making people's sex lives better. We are confident that you will have the same response as our road-test couples—you will be turned on, happier, and closer after 48 hours of trying out this program.

My wife is my number-one priority in life, but I rarely act like it! I tend to get caught up in my work, and that steals time from our relationship. But this weekend I was able to consciously make her my number-one focus, and it was wonderful!

Of course, tastes differ. You might not like as many specific suggestions as we give in this book. Some people like to cook from a recipe; others are just as content to put together a meal from whatever they find in the cupboard. If you're among the latter, you can simply think of the weekend as a special occasion to lavish attention on each other by picking the ideas you like and putting energy and thought into good lovemaking.

Sometimes the weekend can magnify differences in sexual tastes. It's not far-fetched to imagine that some sexual requests will be denied and you may be disappointed. You may experiment and one of you will like it—and want to bring it back to your regular sex life—but the other will say that once was enough. Don't resent your partner for not liking everything you like. If that happens, we suggest that the partner who liked the new activity use it as private fantasy material. The more options you explore, the more likely you are to find new things you both enjoy.

> We needed something like this to remind us of how important we are to each other. Life has a way of distracting you and making you look elsewhere. This program forced us to pay attention to one another, which is something we were both hungry for and didn't even know it.

1

Planning the Setting: Time, Place, and Mood

*Our weekend began as soon as we started reading the book!
We got so turned on, we started planning our weekend immediately. My husband left work early three times during the
week we were planning our trip so we could make love before
the kids got home from school. This was truly unusual; he's
an executive who always works until at least seven o'clock.*

FOLLOW THE PLAY-BY-PLAY INSTRUCTIONS
in this book, and at the very least you'll have a really romantic, erotic, fulfilling weekend. But we're opti-
mistic that this book will do more: You will likely build a
higher level of desire, exploration, and satisfaction into
your sex life by following the program. We provide all the
guidance you'll need, including ideas for sex innovations
and surprises. You make the weekend your own by taking
what you want to customize a sexy romp that suits your
own tastes and schedule. Everything we recommend is
safe, so it's simply a matter of what appeals to you and
your partner, and what you agree to actually try.

Sharing the Planning

Before you begin the weekend program, we strongly recommend that both you and your partner read this book from cover to cover to see what's ahead and what you'll need. We hope that each partner will participate in the planning and preparations. Part of the success of this weekend depends on sharing and team-work. Even if one partner is more motivated to do the program, it's important that each contribute to create a successful weekend. As one partner sees the other cooperating, the mood of emotional generosity is established.

We both took responsibility. We were equally excited about "the project."

We both did the preparation, which was minor. We decided to stay at home and already had most of the stuff we would need.

My wife organized it because her schedule is the tightest; I felt left out. I wished we'd shared this task.

There are exceptions to this rule. If one partner wants to orchestrate the whole weekend to surprise a willing partner by giving the book and sex getaway as a gift, or if one has a partner who would resist a more active role but would enjoy the weekend if everything were provided, it can work with the inspired partner doing all the planning. If these scenarios work for you—and you can do this with pleasure and no resentment—then it's no problem if you read the book, do all the preparation, and make the choices.

> *My husband whisked me off without telling me where we were going. It was one of the most romantic things he ever did.*

> *I was glad my husband hadn't read the book. He had no idea what was coming and was delighted by surprise after surprise.*

SCHEDULING THE TIME

Assuming that both of you are designing this Great Sex Weekend, first you need to agree on a date—maybe a backup date, too—so this *really will* happen. We strongly urge you to devote an entire weekend to the program. If you can manage to dedicate only one day, choose a weekend when you can add on a luxurious Sunday morning. Road-testers were creative in adapting our suggestions to fit their work schedules and budgets. For those who work weekends, taking 24 to 48 hours on weekdays is an obvious and easy adjustment, and some couples reported enjoying lower midweek rates at less-crowded hotels. Some said they are just too tired on a Friday night to get in the right mood, so they started fresh Saturday morning and continued until Sunday night. Others did the same because they could comfortably afford only a single night in a hotel. We loved this commuting couple's solution:

Since we live in two different states, we could manage just one day out of our busy weekends together. But we didn't want to miss anything, so we decided to do one part of the three-day plan on three different weekends. Talk about prolonging the anticipation and pleasure! It worked magnificently.

Discuss a few dates that you know might suit your schedules—for example, a long holiday weekend when you could start the program early and without stress, or a time when business is predictably slow, or during a summer week when the kids will be at camp. You may be tempted to combine the getaway with some other special occasion, like the celebration of a birthday. Some road-testers did that and it worked out well, but we also heard from one couple who had a bad experience because the birthday person expected more attention, and the other felt it was to be a weekend of fair and mutual exchange. And if either of you is a sports buff, think ahead and avoid conflicts with important events.

Suggest a date far enough in advance that you can keep free of other commitments during the scheduled time. (And, women readers, don't forget to consider your monthly cycle, too.) If for some reason you cannot actually agree on a date right now, at least pick a date by which you promise each other you will make a reservation to get away or set a time for an at-home weekend.

GETTING AWAY FROM HOME

We went to the Tropicana in Vegas because they have things you don't get at home or in an ordinary hotel, like mirrors above and beside the bed, dimmer lights everywhere, and an extra-large bathtub.

If you can, we advise you to go away for the weekend. Most road-testers who stayed home said next time they would try to get away. Those people all reached the same conclusion: Your house is full of reminders of things you need to do and other distractions.

Selecting the right getaway location and making reservations is important. Pick a setting that appeals to you both. If she hates rustic places, don't take her to one; if he hates pretentious resorts where everyone is dressed up, find some middle ground. Here are the things you should look for:

The location should be easy to get to. It's a bad idea to start the weekend with any hassle. Don't pick a place that's too hard to find. If a short hop on a shuttle plane takes you someplace romantic, fine, but getting in and out of most airports is an energy drain that detracts from time that could be better spent enjoying the program. In major cities where traffic snarls make driving out of town unpredictable, consider a nice downtown hotel where the service is great and the atmosphere is glamorous.

QUICK TIP #1: Some places may sound romantic but aren't. If you have a friend with a cabin in the woods, find out as much as you can before you go there. A cabin full of creatures or one that hasn't been cleaned in a while is unappealing and may be missing some basic amenities—like a big bathtub—that we suggest you use. However, nice cabins with all the modern conveniences in beautiful settings can also be perfect sites for your weekend.

QUICK TIP #2: In general, we don't recommend bed-and-breakfasts. They can be charming, but most don't offer nearly enough privacy. Consider only those that provide detached cottages, or rooms with thick walls and private bathrooms.

When booking a hotel for this program, make sure your room includes:

- ✩ Both a shower and a bathtub. If bathing together holds appeal, ask if they have any rooms with oversize tubs (extra points for a Jacuzzi).
- ✩ Room service.
- ✩ Bar refrigerators are a plus. (You can always bring a cooler if the hotel offers everything else you want.)
- ✩ Adult movies on pay-per-view or a VCR (so you can bring along your own videotapes). You might consider bringing your own VCR if the hotel does not provide one.
- ✩ Queen-size bed (extra points for a king-size or canopy bed).
- ✩ Charm. Seek a place with out-of-the-ordinary rooms or nice views. (Extra points for a balcony or fireplace.)

QUICK TIP #3: Every hotel has some small, dark, or noisy rooms. Tell the reservation clerk that this is to be a special weekend, and to hold one of the better rooms for you. If you have any doubt, when you get there ask to see a few available rooms before checking in.

> *Tell your readers to ask for a room away from the elevator; we didn't, and the noise detracted from an otherwise perfect weekend.*

> *We always request a room adjacent to a stairwell or an end unit; that guarantees privacy on at least one side of the suite.*

> *I wish I'd asked whether any conventions were going on that weekend. There was one, which made the hotel crowded and detracted from our romantic mood.*

At the back of this book, in the section called "Getaway Places," you will find a selected list of romantic places to stay in or near about two dozen locales in the United States and Canada.

STAYING HOME

If you decide not to travel for whatever reason, you can modify the home setting to ready it for the weekend:

IF YOU CAN AFFORD IT — OR NEED NEW SHEETS anyhow—**we recommend buying new linen for the**

occasion. You can go with tasteful designs for everyday use, or try inexpensive satiny sheets for how differently they feel on this—and future—sexy weekends. (Caution: The satiny sheets may be flammable; keep candles with open flames at a safe distance.) On the other hand, if you worry about stains, you might prefer to put old sheets on the bed, or old towels near the bed. You might even buy a cheap shower curtain or stop at a paint or hardware store and get an inexpensive plastic tarp if you're thinking of trying the body paints. (More about body paints in chapter 5.) At the very least, use fresh sheets for the weekend.

We love flannel sheets to keep cozy in the winter.

A soft cotton throw rug works well for juicy sex.

I bought inexpensive Indian print fabric and draped it over the bed. We pretended we were in a Persian palace!

Lighting is important. Bright, glaring light can make you feel inhibited. A soft, flattering light helps both men and women feel sexy. We sought advice from Marsha Hunt, award-winning writer-producer for *Playboy* Home Videos: "Blue lightbulbs create an atmosphere that is mysterious and sensual. We always use blue light in our bedroom scenes. It gives enough light to see, but it's dark enough to cover flaws, too. Pink bulbs provide light that is very soft, romantic, and flattering (it makes most people look much younger), but stick to a 40-watt bulb if you use pink. Stay away from green—that's monster lighting—and yellow, which makes skin look sallow." We suggest that you stay away from red bulbs, too, because they make the bedroom look like a brothel. You can find blue and pink bulbs at any well-stocked hardware or large discount store.

We decided not to follow your advice and used green light-bulbs, because green is our favorite color and they really helped us feel comfortable and sexy.

I changed our bedside light to pink. It gave the room a soft, romantic feel.

Our road-testers convinced us that the 1960s are fondly remembered—even by those too young to have been a part of the era.

We always find our black light sets a romantic mood; we burn incense too.

We use a blue lava lamp when we make love.

Nothing is as romantic as firelight, so if you have a fireplace, be sure to stock up on firewood. Find a big old comforter to place in front of the fireplace. The delicious smell of wood burning pleases the senses, and you'll have perfect, flickering light for lovemaking.

We hadn't used our fireplace in three years. We spent the entire night in front of it. We had dinner by firelight, and that's where we gave each other our massages. It was incredibly romantic.

We recommend lots of dripless candles—scented if you enjoy that; unscented if scents are distracting. If you have lots of candleholders, pick up a few packages of candles. If you don't have candlesticks, you'll find inexpensive votive candles in glass holders at stores like Pier 1, Target, bath or beauty supply stores, and drugstores; buy at least eight. Banana Republic and Gap now sell nice aromatic candles in containers for a little more money. If you have the space, surround your bathtub with 20 of those short, flat tea lights, the kind packaged in round tins.

QUICK TIP #4: Place all candles on fireproof surfaces, away from drafts. **Never leave any candle unattended.** If you've forgotten candleholders and you're at a hotel, ask for a few ashtrays. If you're in a nonsmoking room, tell them what they'll be used for—management will be happy to help you protect their furniture.

Flowers are always wonderful; they add fragrance, color, and sensual shapes to a room. Especially if you don't usually buy them, flowers announce that it is a special weekend. Buy a bouquet for your dining table or just a stem or two for a bud vase on the nightstand.

I sent flowers to his office as a way to say "I love you." He brought them home for us to enjoy for the weekend.

These were my favorites for the room: freesia, Casablanca lilies, and orange blossoms.

Music is an important part of setting a romantic mood. If you don't already have speakers in your bedroom, move your stereo into the bedroom if it's at all portable. Otherwise, buy or borrow a small boom box or portable CD player that can be used in both the bedroom and the dining area.

Select music that you know you both will enjoy. Play it throughout the weekend, but keep the volume low enough so that you can easily talk to each other—in bed and out.

For this special weekend, try to vary the music you make love to. Sex is different with different kinds of music. For example, if you usually listen to soft mood music, try some light rock 'n' roll. Keeping up with a faster beat can be a lot of fun. If you usually have sex without music, adding music will enhance the experience.

> *Making love to Kitaro, a Japanese New Age artist, is great because there are no words to distract us and the beautiful melodies intensify and prolong our passion.*

> *We started out dancing to Melissa Etheridge but moved to the sofa pretty quickly. Making love to really loud music with a powerful beat is good clean, aerobic fun.*

Think about where you want the VCR. If it's easy to move, consider whether you want it in the bedroom to create a viewing room with maximum comfort.

If your home is not always squeaky clean and free of clutter, invest the time or money for this occasion. Bathtubs, in particular, must look inviting. Reminders of work or house projects should be kept out of sight. If you normally keep lots of pictures of the kids or other family members on the dresser across from your bed, we suggest that you put them away—or at least facedown—so their images don't interfere with the spirit of carefree romance or lust.

DOING THE PROGRAM IN THEIR OWN HOME WAS just right for some road-testers:

> *We love being at home, and we did a lot to make it special. We put the stereo in our bedroom. I always have lots of candles! So I added strings of whimsical lights (we picked out fun and cheap ones from the Lillian Vernon catalog). Little Christmas lights would work, too. I also put lots of flowers everywhere.*

> *Staying at home was great, easy, and we didn't have to spend a lot of money. Friday night we had great finger foods—shrimp cocktail, pot stickers, fried stuffed mushrooms, roasted red pepper and garlic cheese spread on great bread with a good bottle of wine. The next night we got a gourmet pizza delivered.*

> *We just cleaned up, set the candles out, turned the phones off and the soft music on. We were ready to go!*

GUARDING YOUR PRIVACY AT HOME OR AWAY

It is essential to feel that neither your mood nor your activities will be interrupted. Agree to turn off the ringer on *all* phones for the weekend and set the answering machine, if you have one, to its lowest volume so incoming messages don't distract you. If you need to check on the children, elderly parents, or the office via phone or E-mail, set aside one or two specific times during the weekend to make contact with the outside world, and don't violate that schedule.

It's difficult for people with children or other continuous responsibilities to relax unless they know they can be reached for emergencies. We recommend you figure out a way to be "on call" for children or other emergencies, but unreachable by others. For example, if you decide to stay at home and banish the phone, arrange with a trusted neighbor to be your go-between. The neighbor can ring your bell or leave a note on the front door to let you know if you are needed.

Most hotels will agree to block all calls unless the caller states that it is an emergency, or you have given them a list of exceptions. Other calls will be handled by the message service. When considering a hotel, ask if they will provide this service if you think you'll want it. Remember, the best way to be sure no one reaches you is not to reveal where you'll be staying.

Whether staying at home or going away, let friends, coworkers, and relatives know that they can leave a message on your answering machine but that you won't be returning any calls until Monday. Lots of road-testers told friends and family that they'd be out of town when in fact they stayed at home.

A note on child care: If you can't afford a baby-sitter while you're away, perhaps a friend or relative will take care of your young children for the weekend. However, don't leave the children in the care of a neighbor if you're staying at home. The children may not understand why they cannot be with you. If extended family is not nearby and it seems too much of an imposition to leave the kids with friends, think about approaching a couple in a similar situation. Show them the book, tell them a bit about your plans for an intimate weekend, and see if they are interested in swapping child-care favors. They can borrow the book after your weekend, and maybe even some of the items that you bought to enhance your own weekend getaway, then you can arrange to watch their kids. You know the kids will have fun and be safe—and there's no expense.

A note on pet care: Several at-home road-testers were surprised by how much their pets detracted from their weekend hideaway. They all offered the same solution: "Kennel your pets!" If you don't, at least keep them out of the bedroom.

OPTIONAL LONGER-TERM PREPARATIONS

Do I need to diet first? No, don't put off the weekend because you're waiting to reach your "best weight." We live in a culture that idolizes slim, athletic bodies. The challenge for both women and men is to feel desirable even if they aren't at their ideal weight. The slow, sensuous approach toward lovemaking that we suggest makes people feel sexy and turned on. Our motto: If You Think Sexy and Act Sexy, You Will Be Sexy.

If you feel self-conscious about your body, there are things you can do to feel more attractive and comfortable. The low, soft light we recommend not only sets the mood but is flattering. Candles provide the most "generous" lighting effect. We recommend that women who are embarrassed about their extra body weight undress in the bathroom and emerge in a silky, loose-fitting garment (like a dressing gown or oversize man's-style shirt). For those who prefer undressing in front of their partner, wearing a camisole and half-slip makes some women feel slimmer and sexier.

For those who really want to look better before starting the weekend, a short-term, safe, balanced diet and exercise program can make them feel more confident. Such a short regime might only make a few pounds' difference, but that's enough to provide a psychological boost. Even if you don't lose weight, exercise can also firm up your body and make you feel strong, and that will make you feel sexier, too. If your partner is the one who wants to get more fit for you, watching him or her "prepare" is flattering—better yet, do it together.

Do I need new, sexy clothes? We're quite sure that your current wardrobe has everything you need for a sexy getaway. However, buying something new can add to the anticipation of the weekend. Feeling well dressed, especially if your partner is the kind to notice and compliment you on how you look, can make you feel extra sexy. Instead of buying a new outfit for Saturday-night dinner, women might prefer to splurge on lingerie. A black teddy, negligee, or short kimono robe can be arousing for you both—

especially if it's different from what you usually wear to bed.

> *He loves seeing me in sexy lingerie. As a present to him, I bought stockings and a light-blue garter belt with matching bra for me to wear. I had them gift-wrapped and had him open this gift right before dinner Friday night. He couldn't wait to get home.*

If you are planning to buy new lingerie for your sexy getaway weekend, perhaps your partner would enjoy participating. Call the Victoria's Secret catalog (see the back of the book for details on catalogs) and let the anticipation of the weekend build by looking through the catalog and picking out a few items together. Victoria's Secret also sells men's sexy silk boxers, bikini underwear, and kimonos. Initially the man may wear these just to please his partner, but he may soon appreciate how these garments make him feel sexy and attractive, too.

If you are too busy to take a lot of time with these preparations, here's another fun alternative: Take a leisurely trip to a lingerie boutique on the Saturday-afternoon break during your weekend; you'll both look forward to seeing your purchases modeled later that night.

One more thought about clothes: Many women already have teddies or sheer camisoles, and use them strictly as underwear. In the spirit of this weekend, be more adventurous than usual. Wear your teddy under a blazer or suit top instead of a blouse. One of our road-testers suggested another variation on the lingerie theme:

She informed her fiancé that she was wearing no panties under her dress; he rushed her through dinner and back to their apartment for an evening of passionate lovemaking. The power of suggestion should never be underestimated.

We hasten to add that it is not only men who get aroused by sexy underwear or great new clothes. A woman loves to see her man dressing just for her.

> My husband is a jeans kind of guy. He really surprised me by bringing a beautiful suit and tie for our Saturday dinner out. I was flattered that he wanted to look good for me. That was a real turn-on.

Necessary Short-term Preparations

Weeklong Abstinence

The minute we made sex off-limits, we were dying for it.

You wouldn't want to eat a heavy lunch if you knew a sumptuous banquet awaited you that evening. Abstaining for the week before your sexy getaway will heighten your appetite for sexual extravagance. For most couples abstention means giving up one—maybe two—sexual episodes the week before. For others, it will be no sacrifice whatsoever. Our road-test couples confirmed the old axiom that we always want what we can't have. Trying to abstain made them miss having sex more than usual, but they liked the anticipation that was built up for the weekend.

> *The abstinence worked for us. We were really hungry for each other by the time the weekend began.*

> *This was the first time we had to "repress" our desires since the hot, hormonal days of high school.*

> *We abstained for just two nights, and that helped, but a whole week would've added stress for us.*

Another reason for weeklong abstinence has its roots in the therapy program for couples developed by sex researchers Masters and Johnson. Abstaining from genital play shifts the emphasis away from goal-oriented (that is, orgasm-oriented) sexuality to sensuality. You can touch and caress each other. When you and your partner want close contact and want to get beyond cuddling, take turns massaging each other, avoiding the breasts and genitals. Gently knead the little tension knots on your partner's neck, feet, or hands, or massage the head. Very slowly give long strokes down the back, arms, and legs. Getting aroused during the massage is understandable. But a little frustration is going to help create longing and anticipation that serve as a reminder of how much you really desire your partner's touch.

Don't focus just on *getting* pleasure; also notice how touching your partner gives you pleasure, too. Ask your partner to tell you what feels good and what does not. This simple exercise provides a good introduction to learning more about your own body and your partner's body in the week before you embark on the program. Touching all over the body reminds us that we have many erogenous zones besides the obvious ones. If you really want to spend time exploring your own and your partner's sensuality, move Friday night's pleasuring techniques (see pp. 63–64) up to the week before the program.

One additional preparatory exercise will make the erotic mood of the weekend even hotter. Instead of casually undressing in front of each other as usual, be more modest during the week before the program. You can tease each other a bit. Let your partner catch a glimpse of you in sexy underwear, but dress and undress in private. That way you will be especially turned on the first time you take your clothes off in front of each other on the weekend.

> *We added one more rule: We both swore we wouldn't play with ourselves as a way to make the anticipation that much sweeter. I think he held to his end of the bargain. I know I did, and it made me very excited.*

Verbal Foreplay

We know a sex counselor who tells men that if they start verbal foreplay in the morning, their partners will be begging them to have sex that night. The busier your day (hers or his), the more your partner appreciates that he or she is on your mind. If you know your partner can handle it, give fair warning during your verbal foreplay about your hopes that together you will be pushing the boundaries of physical intimacy.

Verbal foreplay should be expressed in your own words. Say only what you mean and say it in a way that fits your style (although you certainly have our blessing to step "out of character" for the weekend). Here are some suggestions that might just get you thinking:

✩ Make a phone call by mid-morning just to say something like "I can't wait until we start our sex getaway tonight." If there are things you've never done before and want to try (new toys, positions, or places), don't keep your ideas a secret. Let your partner experience your anticipation. Knowing that two minds are reviewing the possibilities practically guarantees sexual excitement.

> For a few days before we went on our weekend, I left suggestive little messages on his private voice mail. He loved it.

> My husband called me Friday afternoon, just before our "weekend" was to start, and told me what he was going to do to me—using the present tense, as if it were happening now.

✩ If you prefer the written word, drop a sexy note in a lunch pail or briefcase. Electronic mail can be fun, but it's safest to think of E-mail as a postcard message. If you use E-mail at work, remember that messages get archived and can be retrieved by others. Write something slightly suggestive in secret code that you know your partner—but no one else—will understand. If your E-mail is on a private account, you can afford to be more risqué.

> My husband disguised his handwriting and sent a very romantic letter signed "See you tonight—Your Secret Admirer."

> I dropped off a letter at his shop. He said it really heated him up.

✩   Several women have described "treasure hunts" in which they are the "treasure." One left her lover a note at the front door that led to a pitcher of margaritas, where another sexy note yielded his next clue, and so on, until he reached the "treasure"—his provocatively dressed wife.

> I used an old lipstick to write a countdown on our bedroom mirror the entire week before. He was really excited by the time it read "1 more day."

Communicating Expectations

Everyone experiences this program differently—although the road-testers unanimously reported that seeing the possibilities spelled out ahead of time was enticing and, many added, titillating. Some of those couples had already tried many of the activities we describe, although they confessed they hadn't done some of these things in a long time. Others knew their partner would be "up for anything" and, therefore, had no anxiety suggesting the exercises that they found appealing, even if they'd never done these things before. Nonetheless, some road-testers weren't sure of their partners' reactions about new sexual activities and didn't feel comfortable just coming out and asking for what they wanted. Some were also feeling a little concerned that their partners might want to try an exercise that they themselves were not ready for.

It's perfectly natural to feel somewhat anxious as you anticipate spending such an intimate weekend together.

The best way to reduce pressure and avoid disappointment is to keep an open mind: *Don't expect to do everything we suggest on a single getaway weekend.* This handbook is designed to be used over and over. For couples who are open to experimentation, there are ample suggestions for how to turn up the heat the next time around.

If there's something in particular that you really want to happen—for example, getting or giving much more oral sex than you usually do—you can either wait and see whether the mood of heightened intimacy takes you there naturally, or you can tell your partner ahead of time so he or she can know what's on your mind. In the days leading up to your weekend getaway, take some time to discuss your feelings about particular sexual activities.

> *I overcame my resistance to oral sex when my lover sent me a steamy note that read: "Deep pools of viscous you—I long to go there."*

Several road-testers found discussing sexual interests to be kind of awkward. They felt that they needed help making intimate requests. Happily, a few couples came up with some natural and easy solutions. Our nod goes to the partners who each read the book and highlighted in different colors those exercises and activities that interested them the most. Some even put stars or asterisks in the margins when something really piqued their interest.

> *We each reviewed what we had highlighted. Knowing what the other person wanted got us both excited about the coming adventure.*

I read what she underlined the night before we left. Then we talked about what we were each looking forward to on the way to the motel. That talk was very helpful in setting the mood.

He only skimmed the book. I read it word for word, so in the car on the way down to the hotel we talked about what I wanted to try. It made our commute fun, and he enthusiastically supported my choices.

2

Shop 'Til You Drop
(into Bed)

We had fun shopping for a new bra for the occasion. With both of us in the dressing room "voting" on the best choice, it was a great precursor to a sensual evening.

IN THIS CHAPTER, WE SUGGEST YOU PUR-chase specific items that will enhance your experience. We also indicate where you can find these items easily, least expensively, and, in most cases, with the least embarrassment. (At the back of this book we provide the toll-free numbers to the mail-order catalogs mentioned throughout the book.) We have asked our experts and research assistants for suggestions, and we have also included recommendations from our road-test couples. We've done the planning and legwork so that you can devote your own creative energies to the fun parts of this weekend getaway.

We make lots of suggestions here, and you should simply pick and choose whatever appeals to you. Nothing in this book is required, although several items are highly recommended. Even though shopping for your getaway can be fun, it still takes time. Remember, we believe the weekend works best when each partner takes on some fair share of what needs to be done. Doing some of the shopping for things that you'll enjoy together is one of those gestures that show your willingness to create a truly special time for sex and love.

There are a few ways you can cut corners if you need to save time. First, you don't have to buy a single thing beforehand. You can decide what you want and spend a few hours during the weekend buying the "enhancements" that will make your time together more fun or more sensual. One road-tester adamantly drove home this point:

> *I was too busy to prep—and being too busy is why we needed the weekend in the first place! I relieved my feelings of guilt by suggesting that we shop Saturday afternoon. We bought sexy lingerie, body oils, and candles—that was all we needed to have a great time.*

Second, you may not want to run around being thrifty if you are fortunate enough to have more money than time. Tender Loving Things, Inc., carries many of the products we recommend. Call for information and mention that you are preparing for a Great Sex Weekend. (See appendix 3, "Mail-Order Catalogs.")

For your convenience, we provide a checklist at the end of this chapter. It includes all the accessories you might want for your weekend that we describe in this chapter and in chapter 1.

Highly Recommended Personal Items

These are the few items that we believe will really enhance your weekend experience:

NEW UNDERWEAR. His and hers lingerie are relatively inexpensive teasers. The sexier, the better. Finding sexy underwear for her is easy. If he always wears white Jockey briefs, buy colorful ones. If he always wears long boxers, consider buying the shorter, tighter variety.

LOTIONS AND MASSAGE OILS. These products are easy to find at most shopping malls. Bath stores like The Body Shop and Bath and Body Works carry a variety of scented lotions and oils; they're reasonably priced, ranging from just a few dollars to the costlier natural oils. Well-stocked drugstores and beauty supply shops carry these, too. Just unscrew the caps, take a whiff, and see what you like.

We like the Kama Sutra products—especially the great honey dust powder!

Debra D'Amato, a Beverly Hills masseuse with a celebrity clientele, says that lavender is particularly calming and citrus is uplifting. "Actually, any oil will do," she says. "You can pull out the olive oil or safflower oil from the kitchen cupboard and go for it." She cautions that because all oils stain, you should get out the old sheets and towels so you don't have to worry. She advises that products described as "massage lotions" are less staining than "massage oils," but you still might want to save the satin sheets for another time. Her favorite easily available (it is even sold in grocery stores) lotion is Curél, but any lotion will do. Another word to the wise: Keep oils refrigerated to stay fresh; old oils smell rancid.

SCENTS. Although subtle, many people find smell is an important part of their sexual arousal. We already described how scented candles can add aromatic flavor as well as romantic light to your weekend interlude. You might also want to have on hand some bath oils, bath salts, or bubble bath, nice bars of mildly scented soaps, or the new moisturizing body washes sold with soft, mesh bath "puffs." Some people find the smell of incense overpowering, but others love the erotic aromas of temple incense, lavender, vanilla, raspberry, or gardenia.

Although the aphrodisiac powers of essential oils are not proven, many people believe that certain scents do arouse, among them are jasmine, sandalwood, rose, and ylang-ylang. You can put a few drops in bathwater or mix it with safflower or almond oil to make your own aromatic massage oil.

I love blending scents. Experiment to see what you like. I like burning vanilla and strawberry scented candles together; sometimes I go for cinnamon with vanilla.

LUBRICANTS. These are useful when you are just touching each other during foreplay, and essential for most women when engaging in frequent or prolonged intercourse. Especially if you use condoms, lubricants are needed to keep sex fun rather than irritating or painful. *Never use oil-based lubricants with condoms, diaphragms, or cervical caps because oil causes rubber to disintegrate in a short time.* For condoms or any latex contraceptive barrier, use a water-soluble (glycerin-based) lubricant or one of the new silicone-based ones that last as long as oil but won't harm latex.

The right lubricant can make all the difference in the world. In appendix 3, we describe our favorite brands and where to get them. Some are available in well-stocked drugstores, but others need to be ordered or bought in a specialty store. Astroglide was the first of a class of improved lubricants, but now there are many types that add variety to each sexual experience. Some of these are pricier than the old standards, but worth it.

We spent a year sampling lubes and are happy with our choice—Wet—a light water-based lubricant.

Years ago the "Playboy Adviser" column recommended Albolene liquefying cleanser for those who don't need latex for protection from pregnancy or sexually transmitted diseases, or for the touching exercises that exclude intercourse. You'll find it in drugstores stocked with the other face cleansers, not the lubricants.

*We liked the Albolene gel the best because it was oil based
so it made intercourse feel really smooth and good.*

CONDOMS. If you rely on condoms for birth control
and/or protection from sexually transmitted diseases, be
sure to stock up for the weekend. Buy lots of your favorite
condoms, or use this as an opportunity to be more playful
and buy an assortment, perhaps including lightly ribbed
condoms or other designs that are out of the ordinary. Remember, however, that novelty condoms (like many of the
colored or textured variety) are meant to be gags and
should not be counted on for protection. Also, if you are
considering anal sex, condoms are the best way to protect
the health of *both* partners. See appendix 3 for convenient
mail-order catalogs and Web sites that offer variety packs
for experimentation as well as large quantities of your
favorite condoms at economical prices.

RELAXATION AIDS. We strongly advise couples to
purchase a Happy Massager®—an inexpensive massage
tool. Its five spider-shaped wooden balls (with "happy
face" design) work wondrously to make giving massages
fun and easy on the massager's hands and wrists. Receiving a massage relieves tension and stress, and feels great!
Mark Juarez, inventor of the ingenious Happy Massager®,
says, "Your hands are an extension of your heart. Mutual
massage is important for couples because caring touch—
physical contact that expresses human tenderness—is an
essential component of true intimacy." (See the special
sections at the back of the book for instructions on using

this simple tool, and for how to find names of stores near you that carry the Tender Loving Things line of products, including the Happy Massager®.)

We are also quite fond of Hitachi's Magic Wand, an electric massager found in the small-appliance section of discount houses and large drugstores, along with other brands of massagers; or you can buy one through any of several mail-order sex toy catalogs listed at the back of this book. The difference, however, is that the smooth shape of Hitachi's massage head allows it to serve double duty as a faithful vibrator. For the latter use, we recommend the "slow" speed and starting with a hand towel or pajamas between you and the vibrator until you get used to it.

SEX TOYS. The getaway weekend offers a perfect time to introduce sex toys into your bedroom, or try a new toy, if you already have one or more in your collection. If there's a sex boutique in your city and you don't mind being seen in it, getting ready for your weekend can be almost as much fun as the weekend itself. Sneak away during an afternoon lunch hour or take a more leisurely after-dinner stroll through one of these stores. Just looking at the inventory in stores like Pleasure Chest in Los Angeles or Chicago, New York's Eve's Garden, and San Francisco's Good Vibrations can be an educational experience. Smaller cities have adult novelty boutiques, too.

If there are no stores of this type in your area or if you don't want to be seen in a sex boutique, you can have a catalog sent to your home discreetly. The companies we recommend in this book ship items in plainly wrapped packages. All transactions are strictly confidential, and these mail-order houses *never* sell, give, or trade any customer's name.

> *My wife's parents came to visit, saw our Good Vibrations catalogs, and took one home to order things for themselves.*

An interesting note about who uses sex toys: According to the University of Chicago's recent scientific survey, 16 percent of women and 23 percent of men between ages 18 and 44 find the idea of using sex toys appealing. Another group of sex researchers learned more about those who have actually purchased a sex toy by asking the people who operate the Xandria Collection catalog to send their survey to 1,000 customers. They found that the *typical* person who buys a sex toy is a married, monogamous, college-educated white Christian woman in her thirties—although respondents came from every race, religion (except Muslim), income bracket, and age group. Nearly half were men. Vibrators (both battery and electric) and dildos were by far the most popular toys. The distant third: restraint devices like handcuffs and blindfolds.

> *My husband came up with a clever idea. We didn't want to spend the money on restraints we weren't even sure that we'd like. So he suggested we try his workout "Power Bands" (they're like giant rubber bands connecting Velcro cuffs that were designed to add weight resistance during exercises). Wow! We both found being voluntarily "tied up" was very sexy.*

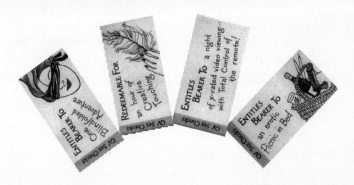

SEX CHECKS. Courtesy of the generous people at Good Vibrations, we have included models of their Sex Checks from its Checkbook of two dozen coupons redeemable for sensual treats. Sex Checks are a way to give your partner the promise of something special, from "Sex in a Semi-Public Place" or an "Erotic Picnic in Bed" to "A Night of X-Rated Video Viewing—with total control of the remote" to "Unlimited Vibrator Induced Orgasms." You can buy books of already printed Sex Checks (see the Good Vibrations catalog in the "Mail-Order Catalogs" section at the back of this book).

We liked the Sex Checks. They did encourage us to do things out of the ordinary. We combined the "Blindfolded Adventure" with the "Oral Pleasure Fest" and really had fun.

I probably would not have introduced my husband to my vibrator without the Sex Check, and he liked it! So I shared my other sex toys with him for the first time—I never had the nerve in the six years we've been together!

NONTOXIC BODY PAINTS. Any well-stocked toy shop or toy department should have a variety of nontoxic paints, including fingerpaints as well as brush-on varieties.

Sight and Sound

PORTABLE SOUND SYSTEM. As stated earlier, music is an important part of setting the right mood. If you plan to go to a hotel, inn, or cabin, take a small boom box or portable CD player with amplified speakers. You can easily borrow this type of equipment if you don't own it. We don't recommend relying on radio fare, since commercial interruptions often take place at the most inappropriate moments.

CAMCORDERS AND POLAROIDS. You may decide to use your camcorder or Polaroid to record some of the sexy moments you'll be sharing. If you're concerned that the videotape or photos may fall into the wrong hands and cause you some embarrassment, plan to destroy them at the end of your weekend.

MUSIC CDS AND TAPES. Well-chosen music not only enhances a romantic atmosphere but the lyrics can provide another way to express sentiments to your partner that you might feel awkward actually saying.

Al Green from the 1970s was the sexiest soul singer ever. He croons with such emotional fervor that his lyrics give me permission to be more open and romantic with my lover.

*We brought several CDs to the hotel that were reminiscent
of our early "insatiable" days.*

VIDEOTAPES. In chapter 5, we offer a range of
choices, from light romantic comedies to sensual R-rated
videos. If you don't own a collection of these, you might
want to head to the video rental store before your weekend begins.

X-rated videos can be both entertaining and arousing.
The better ones can improve your fantasy life as well as introduce ideas for new sexual techniques or settings. However, finding the right adult video takes a little more
thought and planning than finding a good R-rated one.
Bad X-rated videos—those that are too sexist or have too
many gynecological close-ups—are a turn-off. You will
find a list of "Recommended Adult Videos" at the back of
the book.

Feeding the Body—and Soul

FOODS OF LOVE. Have you ever told your partner
that he or she looked good enough to eat? This is the time
to make it happen. There are lots of foods that road-
testers say they like to lick and nibble off their partner's
body: your favorite chocolate sauce, pudding, whipped
cream (some add figs, papaya, or mango, too). Your kitchen
probably has everything you might want, but if there's
some treat that you haven't used in years—or never dared
to try—this is a good time to stock up.

One product we located offers a fun way to express
yourself. Be a sensuous artist with "Tom and Sally's Choco-

late Body Paint," which is handmade with French chocolate (see "Mail-Order Catalogs" at the back of this book). Use the paintbrush included or a cosmetic brush for a softer touch. Delicious on ice cream, too!

SWEET LIBATIONS. If a drink relaxes you and your partner, stock some nice wines and champagnes for the weekend. We also recommend other "romantic" drinks, such as cassis for Kir Royales and good brandies or aperitifs. Hotel bars will serve you festive drinks, but even if you're home, you can pull out a bar recipe book and gather the ingredients for exotic concoctions. It's a lot less expensive to bring your own liquor into a hotel; for wines or champagne, you need only an ice bucket, not a room refrigerator. A few road-test couples mentioned they packed wine coolers for sunset or afternoon picnics. Of course, we caution people not to overdo it: A little liquor helps because it reduces inhibitions, but too much, and there goes the weekend.

In case champagne or sparkling wine is not one of your usual drinks, we have a few recommendations of favorite domestic and imported labels, ranging from inexpensive to the "splurge" zone. In general, we prefer "brut," but those who like sweeter sparkling wines should pick the "extra dry."

Inexpensive ($5–$8)
 Freixenet Cordon Negro (Spanish)
 Paul Cheneau (Spanish)
 Codorniu (Spanish)
 Bouvet brut (French)

Ste. Château Michelle (Washington state)
Korbel (California)

Moderately Priced ($9–$20)
Domaine Chandon (California)
Pommery (French)
Jordan (California)
Mumm's (French)
Mumm's Couvet (California)
Scharffenberger (California Blanc de Blanc Brut)

Expensive ($21–$40)
Moët and Chandon (French)
Piper-Heidsieck (French)
Tattinger (French)
Veuve Clicquot Ponsardin (French)

Splurge (*over* $75)
Cristal (French)
Dom Pérignon (French)

OPTIONAL PERSONAL TOUCHES

EXCHANGING SMALL GIFTS. This is a nice way to start a special weekend with kindness. Gifts are not at all necessary, and many road-testers didn't give them and didn't miss them. We plant the idea just because a little gift can be a great antidote to the brisk and often insensitive pace of everyday life. If you like the idea but it adds to the burden of preparation, wait to buy each other souvenirs during your getaway weekend.

Gift Suggestions

✡ sentimental cards with a few romantic lines that really capture the way you feel about your partner

✡ flowers for her (or him, if he likes them)

✡ a perfume for her or cologne for him that you both find arousing

✡ bath salts or gentle bubble bath

✡ bath sheets

✡ homemade tapes of your favorite music

✡ lingerie (If you've never given a gift of intimate lingerie before, consider it only if you're sure your partner won't consider it crude or embarrassing.)

✡ book of erotic stories. Here are a few recommendations: *On the Wings of Eros: Nightly Readings for Passion and Romance* (Conari Press); *The Mammoth Book of Erotica* (Carroll and Graf); Susie Bright's *Best American Erotica* (Simon and Schuster Trade); Marcy Sheiner's *Herotica 4* (Plume); *Erotique Noire* (Doubleday/Anchor); Lonnie Barbach's *The Erotic Edge: Erotica for Couples* (Plume), and *Slow Hand: Women Write Erotica* (HarperCollins). By the way, if you think erotic readings might add to your weekend, but don't have time to shop, you might go to the popular Web site http://www.nerve.com where you can freely download excerpts from classic and new erotic writing.

Since it was my husband's birthday, I gave him a pair of tight, soft, comfortable fleece pants. He looked so good in them that they definitely helped set the mood.

I sent him flowers. The card in the flowers contained a suggestive poem and I signed off, "Can't wait to pleasure you."

He got silk boxers; I got a CD from my favorite artists.

I bought him flowers and he got me peach bubble bath. These thoughtful gifts got our sex vacation off to a good start.

I bought him a card. My husband liked it but said, "Let's get to the sex!"

GIFTS TO AVOID. Anything expensive. This weekend is about focusing on each other, not material goods. Besides, an expensive gift might make your partner worry about expectations or feel bad if his or her gift to you isn't extravagant. Not all our road-test couples followed our advice; however, we assume this wife wasn't upset:

I had flowers sent to the room so they'd be waiting for her. Then I told her there was one more surprise somewhere in the room. I had slipped a heart-shaped pendant under one of the pillows. When she finally found it, I dropped down on one knee and asked her to marry me all over again. Any other time, I would've felt silly. This weekend I gave myself permission to be all-out romantic, and she loved it.

The Great Sex Weekend
Checklist and Shopping List

___ snacks for the trip and in the hotel room

___ bed linens

___ colored lightbulbs

___ firewood

___ scented candles/candleholders

___ flowers

___ cards/notes

___ new lingerie

___ body lotions/massage oil

___ scented soaps or body wash

___ bath salts/bubble bath/bath oils

___ lubricants

___ condoms, spermicide, or other contraceptives

___ Happy Massager® (wooden tool)

___ Hitachi Magic Wand (electric massager)

___ sex toys (vibrator, Sex Checks, etc.)

___ body paints

___ CDs or tapes (and the portable sound system on which to play them)

___ adult video (for purchase or rental)

___ romantic comedy video

___ chocolate sauce or other "body" food

___ champagne, wine, or other alcohol

___ personal gifts

3

Friday Night

The anticipation of starting our weekend created an aura that was visible to my friends, several of whom remarked that I was glowing.

I T'S FRIDAY AND YOUR WEEKEND IS ABOUT to begin. Do whatever it takes not to be distracted by work or family obligations. If you can, leave work early. If you have kids, get them into the care of a baby-sitter directly after school. Give yourself time to make a mental transition, finish your packing, and make final preparations. Your goal is to have everything taken care of by dinnertime.

If you're staying at home, make a last-minute check of food, flowers, bath and massage oils, and other items you've included from our suggestions in the preceding chapter. Place the candles throughout the house. Hide all vestiges of work. Make the bed look inviting. Put fresh flowers by the bedside and/or in the bathroom. If you feel like it, spray the rooms with a gentle perfume. Burn some mild incense to introduce an exotic scent like eucalyptus or magnolia to evoke a mood of sensuality, seduction, and romance.

If you're going to a hotel, review your checklist before you depart. It's a good idea for one of you to call ahead to make sure the room is the one you've requested. Minimize the possibility of disappointment. When you check in, set up your candles, portable sound system, flowers, and anything else you brought to set the atmosphere and personalize the room.

You may feel ready to make love as soon as you enter the bedroom. We suggest holding back. You'll want to build more tension and anticipation. Shower or bathe by yourself.

Make your bath luxurious by adding rose water or scented bath oils. If you feel like it, turn yourself on a bit by touching your body slowly, gently exploring your genitals until you feel the beginnings of desire. But save yourself for your partner.

If you're hoping or expecting to have oral sex later in the evening, make sure you're very clean. A good wash, using a mild glycerin soap, can make all the difference in a partner's enthusiasm. With this type of soap, a woman can insert a soapy finger up to the first knuckle to cleanse herself inside as well as out. Some women like to shave the pubic hair away from the vaginal lips so that less odor is kept in the pubic area. If the man is uncircumcised, he needs to take special care to clean beneath the folds of the foreskin. Both men and women can add a bit of interest by dabbing their body with a great scent.

When you dress, change privately. Act as though you are getting ready for a date. A woman can dab perfume or cologne in sensual places like the back of her neck or between her breasts. If he or she has strong preferences, check ahead for what scent most arouses desire, or use one that was a present from your partner.

It's always nice to surprise the senses in unexpected ways. If you dare, wear sexier underwear than you normally choose. Some women like to wear an old-fashioned garter belt. Or, if it turns you or your partner on, wear no underpants at all. Do whatever makes you feel sexier—maybe even a little naughty—and what you think your partner would appreciate.

> *I wore fishnet stockings under my dress and no underwear. It was freezing that night in Denver, so I suffered a bit for my surprise—but it was worth it!*

NOW YOU'RE READY TO START THE PROGRAM. Keep our guiding principle in mind: Everything is optional. There isn't time to do it all. We have rated some activities "highly recommended," but do the exercises that appeal to both of you. We arranged the exercises to achieve maximum effect, but this is not a military manual. You may wish to reverse order, skip around, move activities from one day to the next, and so forth. What's important is to relax, have fun, feel close, and lavish the kind of attention on each other that you did in the early days of your relationship.

EXERCISE 1: *An Early-Evening Walk*

Fresh air always raises our spirits. Walking, even in the rain, felt invigorating, intimate, and refreshing.

Take a leisurely walk for about a half hour. It's time to talk a bit. Emotional intimacy helps create physical intimacy. However, be careful about the subject matter. Your conversation should be lighthearted and romantic rather than anxiety provoking or a reminder of responsibilities left behind. Avoid discussing children, bills, work, or anything that can make you worry or feel anxious. Here are some ideas:

- ✰ Reminisce about your first days spent together. Share what you each remember about first impressions, feelings after the first few meetings, what each one of you said during your first few phone calls, significant early events, and when you each knew you were in love.
- ✰ Recall the first time you had sex. What were your feelings at the time? What do you remember most affectionately about your experience or the first morning that you woke up together?
- ✰ Remember your wedding—the preparations for it, the funny parts, the best parts. Together re-create your wedding night, scene by scene.

After our walk, we went home and opened our wedding album from 14 years ago. We hadn't looked at these for a long time. It made us feel very close.

We brought the videotape from our commitment ceremony to the hotel. We hadn't seen it for years, so it was great to reminisce.

☆ Tell each other what you like most about each other. Surprise your partner by sharing traits that you find endearing. Tell your partner about qualities you take the most pleasure or pride in about yourself.

We talked about how our sex life had been on hold for a while and how we really need to work on it. We also talked about music and what we liked. He told me how beautiful I was.

Dinner Interlude

If you choose to dine out, find a restaurant that will provide the most romantic atmosphere, with attractive lighting, enough space between tables for real privacy, and quiet enough to hear each other talk. If room service is your preference, eat by candlelight. If you're having dinner at home, make it a treat. Put out your best china and glasses and, if you have a small table that can be moved easily, consider dining in front of the fireplace, or on a balcony or porch. If you prefer being more casual, have a picnic with fancy paper plates in front of the fireplace or in the backyard. Make it romantic. Light the room with candles; place a small flower next to each plate. Use your imagination to make the dinner as appealing to the eye as it should be to the taste buds. If you're not confident of your own cooking skills, order in a "gourmet" meal . . . anything but the standard Chinese takeout or pizza.

We grilled chicken outside in the middle of a snowstorm and then came inside and cuddled by the fire. It was very romantic.

Whether eating out or in, we recommend a light meal. Passion can get thwarted by a full stomach. Plan to have other special foods on hand later in the night, after you've worked up your appetite again. We suggest making a meal of a series of grazing foods, such as several appetizers for a variety of taste treats, or splitting an entrée. Finger foods always have a nice sensual feel and look to them: grapes and other kinds of small fruit, melon wrapped with ham or prosciutto, artichokes, cut vegetables with unusual dips. Think of this meal as foreplay.

I roasted a bulb of garlic and with my fingers smeared it on thin slices of a sweet baguette with herb brie cheese and a touch of mango chutney, and fed it to her.

Road-test couples have suggested simple dishes like angel hair pasta with just an oil and basil and tomato sauce that isn't too rich. Warning: If either of you is sensitive to strong odors, stay away from foods with lingering smells (like fish, garlic, or onions). One road-test couple remarked that they both smelled like smoked salmon all night and "it kind of broke the mood." If possible, fix things that can be prepared ahead of time. This way you can feel like a guest at your own party.

It's wise to be cautious about alcohol. Be especially careful if you know you're a lightweight drinker. If alcohol is one of life's great pleasures to you, you can have more toward the end of the evening, or perhaps some port wine to have with dessert.

Dinner Talk

It was fun to have suggested topics to talk about. We made it a game to propose topics we'd never thought about before.

Here are a few topics for dinner conversation, or continue the subjects described earlier that you didn't have time to explore during your walk:

- ☆ A dream vacation: Even if it's years away, plan its basic shape. Where would you both like to go? What type of accommodations would be ideal? How long would you want to stay away?
- ☆ Reminisce in detail about the best vacation you ever took together. What made it so special?
- ☆ Take turns describing the things you like about the way your partner makes love to you.

We really enjoyed all the talking exercises. We got to thinking, remembering, and sharing with each other; these were the most intimate moments we had had in a long time.

During your intimate dinner, touch hands, or discreetly graze a breast or a thigh. A little shoeless footwork under the table is always nice, too. A few short but soulful kisses set a nice mood. Stay in your personal comfort zone for public displays of affection, but be flirtatious with each other. A little exhibitionism can be a turn-on if you both like it.

EXERCISE 2: *Undressing Each Other*

That first night, maybe the sexiest thing she did was to undress tantalizingly and slowly.

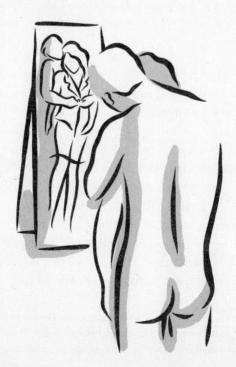

A recent survey revealed that both men and women found watching a partner undress to be as appealing sexually as receiving oral sex. That doesn't mean everyone likes to be watched while undressing. Still, if you can stand the scrutiny, it is usually very sexy to slowly and flirtatiously strip for your partner. Or if it would make you less self-conscious, take time and undress each other. It doesn't matter who starts. Take turns taking off one piece of clothing at a time. Do it slowly. Do it to turn each other on.

Try this variation while standing up. With a light touch, as you take off your partner's shirt or blouse, trace your fingers around his or her chest, breast, nipples. Let the clothes fall where they may. Don't worry about anything but each other. Be as tender and delicate as possible.

EXERCISE 3: *Kissing*

We don't spend enough time kissing. When we really concentrated on it, things started to heat up.

Kissing is very important. Women's number-one sexual complaint is that they don't get kissed enough. But this is an easy problem to fix. Pretend that this is your first experience kissing. Remember this is your "first time," so you probably won't be in the bed. You're not sure what your partner will like. Be tentative and exploratory. You can kiss with a closed or open mouth; with or without tongue; light, medium, or hard. Start out with the lightest approach possible—kissing the lips, cheek, forehead, ears, and throat. Then kiss on the lips a little harder. Use medium pressure with the mouth closed and, again, with

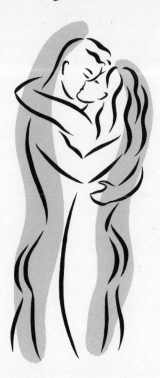

the mouth slightly open. Now kiss with the mouth more open and your tongues touching. You might punctuate these deep kisses with a little nibbling, especially if you know your partner likes that. Talk about what you each liked best, and use those kisses for the rest of the evening.

We pretended that we were strangers kissing for the first time. Delicious.

We giggled and couldn't do this exercise the first time we tried it. But we tried again when we were really turned on, and then it was fabulous.

Of course, this isn't really the first time you've kissed, so one or both of you might feel a little silly—even laugh. That's understandable. It's always good to have fun in bed. However, if only one of you seems amused, and the other is serious, don't take it as a sign that the amused partner doesn't want to do the program. Just kiss longer and differently than usual before moving on to your next exercise.

EXERCISE 4: *Pleasuring*

The touching exercises helped me find places on my husband that I would never have thought to be erogenous zones—like the backs of his knees.

Pleasuring is a highly recommended technique some therapists use to slow down the rush to intercourse and concentrate on sensuality. It also helps people rediscover the full range of erotic stimulation. Pleasuring involves exploring the body to test every possible part of the body for sensitivity before any conventionally erotic zones can be touched. Erotic pleasuring is allowed everywhere except *inside* the body.

You and your partner should take turns throughout this exercise, giving a few minutes to each body area described below. Linger longer if you're both really enjoying it. Move your fingers much more slowly than usual to increase the intensity for both of you.

☆   Start at the toes. Touch your partner's toes lightly using one or a few fingers, then caress the toes and feet with your whole hand. Ask your partner what feels good.

☆ Move up the leg, touching ankles, calves, and inner and outer thighs—first with the light touch, then harder. Keep asking for feedback; the person being touched answers with "That's great," or "That tickles," or "Harder, please." If you are responding, be sure to say "That's perfect" or "Just right" when it is.

☆ Now start on the back. Concentrate on the buttocks, then move up to the lower then upper back and neck. Massage the hairline, head, and earlobes. Ask for a response.

☆ Now move to the front, but skip the genitals for now. Lightly touch the stomach, chest, and nipples; you can use more pressure on the front shoulder area. Continue to talk about how every part of the exercise feels.

What turned him on the most was when I lightly touched his entire body with the front of my fingernails.

If you're really enjoying this exercise, you can start all over with substituting light kisses, licking, or sucking on some of the body parts declared "sensitive." This time move from top to bottom. Or move right into the next exercise.

If you already did this exercise during the week of preparation, you may want to give each other short gentle massages using the Happy Massager® or exchange full-body massages, described in chapter 5.

EXERCISE 5: *Eye Contact*
(*Highly Recommended*)

The most erotic experience was practicing eye contact Friday night. We usually close our eyes and give in to the feelings during foreplay. But looking at each other again really heightened the intimacy.

It has been said that the eyes are the windows to the soul. According to sex therapist David Schnarsch, eyes are also the gateway to intimacy, and most couples deny themselves greater intimacy because they do not look at each other during lovemaking. Take a few minutes and, while touching each other, look into each other's eyes and draw out the trust, emotion, and vulnerability that exist between you. If you feel like you have to look away, do so, but try to return each other's gaze as much as possible. We will want you to repeat this exercise during intercourse later in the weekend, so you need to start practicing better eye contact now.

MOVING TOWARD ORGASM

We held off from orgasm. Bringing each other almost to climax but making each other wait only intensified the experience when we finally let each other go.

We fully expect that after a week of abstinence, most of you will want an orgasm on Friday night—but we encourage you to hold off on intercourse until the following day. Tonight you can get back to serious petting in a way that probably characterized the earliest days of your sexual exploration. This is not just for the sake of nostalgia, but it slows things down, allowing you to rediscover each other's body. It's a break from "same old, same old," and will also heighten passion and appreciation of intercourse when you finally indulge on Saturday morning.

> *Having to abstain from intercourse really brought us together. We did other things to please each other. When we finally had it, we really appreciated it and our response was much more intense.*

We want you both to have great orgasms. Below we describe a variety of ways to be satisfied. We think talking to each other can help. Just as in the pleasuring exercise, continue telling each other what feels good, where you'd like more or less pressure, how turned on you are, or anything else you'd like to say!

OPTION: *Touching the Genitals*
One way you can explore the way your partner likes to be touched is to watch your partner touch him- or herself. This isn't for everyone, but you can learn a lot about your partner's preference for pressure, rhythm, and technique if he or she is willing to show you.

If you prefer to touch each other simultaneously, while gazing and exchanging feedback as well as kissing, that's up to you. If you do that, we do not recommend trying for simultaneous orgasms, because the idea here is pleasure without pressure. Each person should take a turn pleasuring the other to orgasm. You'll learn more about your partner's orgasmic response if you are not simultaneously wrapped up in your own.

> *I think it's important just to have* my time *and* your time. *You can't touch the person giving pleasure. Then it's great when you switch.*

If you've been reading ahead, you know tomorrow is Sadie Hawkins Day, when we encourage women to pleasure their men first. So if you are going to take turns tonight, it's a good time to be chivalrous and apply the "ladies first" principle to who gets the first orgasm of the weekend. Besides, women often complain that many male partners don't give them enough attention. If the man comes first, he might get sleepy; his preorgasmic state of arousal will keep him awake so he can lavish attention on her orgasm.

Of course, not all women have orgasms, or have them regularly, and some men have trouble climaxing every time. In this case, just enjoy the exercises and don't put pressure on yourselves. Being less goal oriented switches the focus to sensuality, which is quite pleasurable even if you don't have an orgasm.

OPTION: *Touching Her to Orgasm*
When you are touching her, practice your eye-contact exercises. Don't forget to smile, kiss, and fondle other

parts of her body every so often. Trace your fingers on the insides of her thighs (checking to see if this feels good or if it tickles). Let her feel how you are totally absorbed and taken with her. Start stroking her labia very, very gently. Ask her if she would like anything harder or softer. Remember, this is not lovemaking as usual. You are rediscovering her body. Tonight marks a change of pace from the usual routine. So ask her every so often about rhythm and where and how hard she wants to be touched.

Gently put two fingers inside the lips on each side of the clitoral shaft, and trace the opening around the clitoris; you can *gently* squeeze the clitoris between your fingers. Don't put a finger inside or on the clitoris for any length of time until everything is quite wet. You can wet your finger by putting it in your mouth or you can use a small amount of lubricant, if needed. Then slowly penetrate with a finger while using the other hand to very gently touch around the clitoral area, asking her if she wants you to touch the clitoris directly or just around it. Ask her what she likes. Tell her about your own excitement to help build her enjoyment and passion.

My partner touched me very slowly, gently, and really explored my whole genital area. I felt like he didn't miss touching anything. It was very sensual and ultimately made me extremely turned on.

Be slow, patient, and luxurious with your fingers. Be consistent when erotic tension is mounting. Sometimes when women get close to orgasm, they lose the climax if anything—the rhythm, the area being touched, the strength of pressure—changes. When she seems close to orgasm, ask her to tell you (whisper, full voice, scream—whatever) if she wants you to keep doing what you're doing. That way there's no mistaking what she wants, and she'll have enough confidence to go over the edge to an ecstatic orgasm.

OPTION: *Giving Her Oral Sex to Orgasm*

We decided to use sliced fruit in small pieces and rub them on our genitals. We also kept a little in our mouths while we were having oral sex.

If you are adding oral sex, go down on your partner after you have stimulated her with your hand. If she is on her back, begin by kissing her and whispering endearments. If she feels self-conscious, tell her how much you love touching her and how much you want to be between her legs, tasting her juices and feeling her tension mount under your tongue. Make her feel confident by telling her that she is giving you erotic pleasure, too.

Many women can achieve orgasm through oral stimulation only when they feel safe, comfortable, and desirable. Some women may feel inhibited because they fear that their genitals are somehow unpleasant to taste or smell. If it takes a woman a long time to climax, she may get concerned that her partner is getting tired or bored, or worse yet, will stop just before her orgasm. Be thoughtful: Let her know that you are comfortable, that she tastes good, and that she can take as long as she likes. The vast majority of men—nine out of ten, according to one major survey—say they enjoy giving oral sex to women. It's a great turn-on if she really believes you are very aroused and into giving her pleasure.

The verbal feedback introduced in the pleasuring and touching exercises is now more important than ever. A woman who wants to be sure that her partner doesn't change anything when she is on the verge of climax needs to say, "Yes, that's it," or "Oh, yes, right there," or "I'm going to come soon."

Partners should know that the whole genital area can be very sensitive and almost anything will feel good once a woman is fully aroused. Take lots of time to explore her with your mouth. Gently lick and suck on the entire area—the vaginal lips, the clitoris, as well as the area above and below it (the small area between the vaginal area and the anus can be very erotic). Alternate sucking and licking, and keep asking what she likes most. If you can, keep touching her with both hands. Use them to reach up and gently massage her breasts or tug lightly on her nipples. Unless you know your partner likes her breasts to be grasped roughly—or she tells you to do that—use a light touch. Or caress her breasts with one hand while you use the other to penetrate her vagina with one or more fingers. If she's really excited and relaxed, this is going to feel fabulous.

OPTION: *Anal Stimulation*

If you know she enjoys anal stimulation or she's indicated that she would like to try it for the first time on this weekend, you can rub the anus externally, or, with a lot of lubricant, gently penetrate it with the tip of one finger. Slowly move the tip of the finger in and out. Ask her if that feels good. If she likes it, move the finger in a little farther (make sure your nails are filed and short). If she's not sure, or says no, don't try it again during this session unless she asks for it. **Be cautious. If you have touched the anal area, thoroughly wash your hands before touching her vagina again. You don't want to transfer bacteria from one area to another.**

OPTION: *Touching Him to Orgasm*

With the man on his back, start gently stroking his penis. A light lubricating lotion can be used if he likes the feel of it. The entire penis has nerve endings, but the areas most sensitive to touch are the glans (the head of the penis), the corona (the ridge of the glans), and the frenum (the strip of skin connecting the glans to the shaft on the underside of the penis). Gently trace the fingers across these areas, then down the shaft of the penis. Gently put the penis shaft between your thumb and your forefinger (or use the thumb and two or three fingers) and apply gentle but firm pressure while stroking it. Ask your partner how much pressure he likes, and if he wants one hand on the shaft or would prefer you put it between both. Ask him how he feels until he tells you what you are doing is just right.

When the shaft feels dry, and if you are not going on to oral sex, use your saliva or lubricant and put it on the shaft so your hand glides. Let your hands slide over the head of the penis and gently touch under the ridge again. Ask if the pressure is right; ask if the rhythm feels good. Modify both according to his requests. Ask your partner if he wants his testicles touched, and if so, how. Many men like to have their testicles lightly stroked or cupped.

OPTION: *Giving Him Oral Sex to Orgasm*

A lot of men say their most intense orgasms take place during oral sex. This may be the case for your partner, and you may want him to climax this way tonight. If you like giving him that pleasure, tell him what you are about to do and how much it excites you to do it. This will turn him on more.

If neither partner has much experience with oral sex, this would be a good time to experiment. But don't force it. This is true for both partners. If unequal desire for oral sex has been an issue between you, don't make it an issue tonight. Perhaps come back to this option tomorrow when more experimental urges might prevail. Or let your partner know that you might be ready to try this next time you use this book for a weekend getaway.

If you decide to have oral sex, take it slowly and easily to begin with, and take a break if you feel tired or uncomfortable. You can relax your jaw by alternating sucking with licking the highly sensitive parts of the penis. This should be a turn-on for both partners. Giving oral sex for too long can become more of a chore than a pleasure to many women, so do it as long as it gives you both enjoyment.

There are easy ways to perform oral sex that will give pleasure to him and to you. Put your mouth over the head of the penis and slowly lick the head, the underside of the ridge, and the shaft. Then begin sucking, gradually adding more suction and checking every so often how much pressure he likes. When you think you understand how much suction is pleasing to him, also ask how hard or fast you should be touching him. Then slowly take more of the shaft into your mouth, keeping suction going, until you have as much as you can handle comfortably. Vary the intake by taking in a little, then a lot. If he gets close to orgasm, encourage him to talk to you, yell, whatever. Grab his buttocks with each hand and pull him to you. Do this with steady motion until he says he's about to come. Continue if you want him to ejaculate this way, or stroke him to his finish if you don't want him to climax in your mouth. He'll enjoy it either way, and watching him ejaculate can be really sexy for both partners.

We suggest partners share responsibility for each other's pleasure. Take turns pleasuring yourself with a hand while your partner licks and sucks around your genitals.

OPTION: *Anal Touching for Him*

Ask him if he would like you to touch his anus. Or you might just put your finger there to stimulate the exterior of the opening, then ask if he likes the feel of it. Some men like penetration by one or more fingers. Ask him if he would like to try. If so, make sure you have plenty of lubrication on your finger. Make sure your nails are filed and short.

If you both are monogamous and your health status is absolutely confirmed, you can do this without a latex finger covering; however, some people don't like the idea of putting an uncovered finger up the anus. If finger cots (they look like tiny condoms) would help you get over your inhibitions, by all means get some at a sex shop, drugstore, or medical supply store. Ease your finger in a little bit at a time, maybe just a fingertip for the first time. If the man is tensing up, don't push. If he is relaxed, you'll feel it and be able to slide in easily.

It is best not to try this before the man is intensely turned on. Even so, anal stimulation may do nothing at all for him. If he says he doesn't like it, stop and don't try it again this session. You can always discuss it later to find out if he'd ever like you to try it again.

On the other hand, some men and women who are doing this for the first time will be surprised how much a man can enjoy this, especially when he is extremely excited and his penis is being stimulated manually or orally at the same time. Put your finger by his anus when he is getting close to orgasm, moving it in and out slowly and carefully. The combination of the finger, your mouth, your hand, and your sounds will ensure that he'll have one incredible orgasm.

INTERCOURSE TO ORGASM

It was exciting to know that our kissing and foreplay would not immediately lead to intercourse. More time was spent exploring, and it forced us to continue our other activities.

Then, when intercourse did come, it was overwhelming. You don't take anything for granted if it isn't always available.

After a week of abstinence, some couples will prefer to do abbreviated versions of the above exercises just as foreplay, and save their orgasm for intercourse. If you do want intercourse, pick any position that you both enjoy. If only one person has had an orgasm or has been sexually satisfied by touching or oral sex, make sure this time is tailored to the partner who prefers to have an orgasm during intercourse. Or you both may have delayed orgasm until you could enjoy it during intercourse.

I started touching him while saying let's not do it until tomorrow. I said it to get him crazy, but I was just teasing. No way I was waiting any longer. I wanted him inside of me tonight.

After Orgasm

Often, men and women have different approaches to post-orgasmic moments. Some men are guilty of rolling over and going to sleep or, worse yet, reaching for the television remote control. Some women are accused of being insatiably interested in conversation. For this special weekend, let's play by women's rules. These few days are about special treatment.

So, after orgasm, take a few moments to express affection. Avoid criticism; you can talk about the specifics at another time. Then, if possible, order up room service or go get a glass of dessert wine, or champagne, or hot chocolate, if that's your thing. Consider having dessert in bed or a midnight snack if you are suddenly ravenous. Unless you're having room service, prepare your little feast together. Have your late-night food and drink and cuddle for a while.

If you are still feeling awake, suggest short (five minutes long) reciprocal massages to help you relax. Since it's too late to do a full-body massage, just concentrate on the feet, hands, and head. Or just the upper shoulders and neck. Consider it one last delicious gift to each other before you have a nice sleep. Don't set the alarm. And if one of you wakes up during the night and reaches over, don't discourage it. More intimacy is fine if you're both interested.

4

Saturday Morning and Afternoon

We like sex in the morning. We wake up together and we feel more rested, more sensuous, and then we can make it as long or as short as we like.

Waking up Together

Sleep in Saturday morning, and when you get up remember to be extra affectionate. You are having an affair with each other this weekend. The mood is romantic and out of the ordinary. Kiss, snuggle; don't just jump out of bed. But don't get *too* affectionate. We don't want you to make love just yet.

The order of activities this morning really should be determined by circumstance and preference. If you wake up famished, breakfast will have to be first on your agenda. But maybe you'd prefer to lie in bed for a while and use the Happy Massager® on each other now, rather than later in the morning. Some people may feel they need to bathe before any more sexual activity, while others who wake up aroused will obviously prefer making love first, and plan to shower and have breakfast later. Do what feels right to you. **Think of the following recommendations as recipe ingredients that can be added in any order.** We offer one plan for the morning that we know worked well for the road-test couples who tried it.

> We liked relaxing in bed. We woke, talked, massaged and pleasured each other. Although we didn't have intercourse, we did make love to each other.

Breakfast in Bed

We recommend breakfast in bed as one way to maintain the weekend's warm and sensual feeling. If you are in a hotel, order up something special like a mimosa (orange juice and champagne) with your food. If you're at home, breakfast can be both luxurious and simple—perhaps croissants with a poached egg on a pretty plate, or just warm scones, coffee, and juice. You can make a half melon more tempting by filling it with ripe berries. Unless cooking is part of foreplay for you, don't interrupt the flow of the morning by having to spend too much time in the kitchen.

Special note for those of you at home: One of you can make and serve breakfast on Saturday and the other person can do the honors on Sunday. Put together a nice tray. For example, include a vase with a flower in it and slice exotic fruit—like mango, papaya, or kiwi—on a plate. Use cloth napkins. Anyone will appreciate these thoughtful touches. Be careful not to ruin the mood by bringing up everyday worries and responsibilities as part of breakfast conversation. Forget about the dishes, if you can. Today, show that you are eager to get started on the next phase of the getaway program.

> *My husband cooked us a breakfast of eggs Benedict and served it to me in bed. He is a good cook and usually shows his love and appreciation through cooking.*

> *We made breakfast together and went back to bed. It was more fun for us to do it together.*

> *We used the leftover fresh fruit from our breakfast for our fun in bed.*

BATHING TOGETHER

> *After we were both soapy, we put our arms around each other and moved our bodies up and down against each other very gently. The feel of gliding bodies is very sensual.*

The first order of the day is to take a sensual shower together. If you like, use an invigorating loofah sponge or soft-mesh cleansing puff on each other. Have on hand a few special scented bar soaps that smell of vanilla, strawberry, papaya, gardenia—whatever pleases you. Let all your senses participate in this shower. Make it feel exotic and sexy.

Take turns soaping each other up. Take your time and pay attention to each part of your partner's body. Massage the shampoo into his or her hair, using your fingers to knead neck and shoulders, too. Does he or she want more or less pressure? *Practice asking for and giving feedback all weekend long*. Once your partner is in a state of pleasure meltdown, move your hands over the rest of the body, starting from the top down. Let your hands linger on each other's chest, breasts, lower back, and legs. When you touch the genital areas, touch to arousal but don't get carried away. Be careful about where you put soapy fingers. If you put them inside the vagina or anus, the soap might sting.

After you're all soaped up, take turns slowly rinsing each other's hair. Kiss each other with the water dripping down your face. Run the hot water over two washcloths and gently apply them to the neck, genitals, or anywhere else that a little added warmth might feel good.

After you dry off, go back to bed in your towels or, if you prefer, put on some new lingerie or bedclothes that you bought just for this weekend. Try to notice your partner's change of appearance and be admiring. Part of what makes us feel sexy is hearing how great we look.

Theme for the Day: "Sadie Hawkins Day"

Loved it! It gave me permission to be aggressive, and he could relax since he did not have the responsibility to initiate.

Speaking from the male perspective, I am definitely more turned on when my partner initiates intimacy.

From after breakfast to just before dinner, all physical and sexual overtures are to be initiated by the female. (*Note to all couples*: Whichever partner initiates sex less frequently should be the one who takes the initiative for this part of today. In most relationships, that's the woman, but if this is not the case in your situation, then have the man initiate.)

I initiate 99 percent of the time when we have sex. I am usually the one who takes control of our sex. So my husband needed to be the initiator on Sadie Hawkins Day.

While most men are used to being the sexual initiator and enjoy it, always being the one responsible for sex can also be a burden and poses the risk of rejection. Most men don't get to explore the side of their personality that might like being guided through a sexual encounter that was shaped by someone else's imagination or pacing. Also, men often express the wish to be desired. When his partner "takes over," a man knows how much she wants him—

but apparently this doesn't happen often enough. Surveys have shown that infrequent initiation of sex by women is men's number-one complaint about what's wrong with their sex life.

Unfortunately, women have been warned away from sexual leadership—even in long-term relationships. Women have traditionally been trained not to be too aggressive with male partners. Many women and men see aggressive moves as unfeminine, too demanding, or threatening to the male's sense of control. Some women have had male partners who reacted badly to their sexual overtures. It's true, in fact, that most men do not want to feel sexually dominated the majority of the time, but it's also true that many would like to be overpowered every now and then. Women get to enjoy feeling "irresistible," so why shouldn't men? We are going to encourage women to experiment with a little sexual dominance just to see how erotic it can be.

I undressed him in front of a mirror, taking my time with each button, touching his nipples under his cotton undershirt, which is a sensation I love. I lingered over the belt and the zipper. We both started breathing more heavily right then.

To start, the woman should get ready to undress her man, any way she wants. She can ask him to undress slowly while she watches (be sensitive to whether or not this would be fun for him or too embarrassing) or she can undress him herself. He then lies down on the bed and she gives him a short but stimulating back massage with the Happy Massager®, that wonderful gizmo described in chapter 2 that makes massage easy to give and lovely to receive. (See the simple instructions we include in the Happy Massager® Guide at the end of the book to show you where and how to use it.) A few minutes with the Happy Massager® is a sweet gift from one partner to the other that feels great while not requiring too much strength or energy. After she has massaged him, he should return the favor.

When you are both feeling cared for, lie facing each other, hold each other, and talk about how you would like to make love. If it doesn't matter to him, she should decide on a position for intercourse, like the ones illustrated later in this chapter. The female partner should start the touching, or she should ask how her partner wants to be touched and explain how she wants to be touched. Remember, this weekend is all about a revitalization of communication skills. Don't take anything for granted or assume you know what your partner wants at that moment. Even if soft stroking is usually preferred, at this moment he or she might want something stronger or lighter or focused on a specific area. It's okay to say "keep touching my breasts" or "move your hand faster " or "suck me a little, softly." Express whatever it is you would really like to have.

He blindfolded me during the foreplay. That intensified the feelings.

When both of you are really aroused, the female partner moves herself into one of the positions for intercourse.

We would like you to consider trying at least one, and perhaps all four, of our suggested alternative positions for lovemaking. Even if you end up in your usual position—whatever that is—make sure you also try something new or a position you use less often than others.

Exotic Option for Birth Control

You might try to do something new if you use a barrier method of birth control. Since this is Sadie Hawkins Day, it is up to the woman to suggest this. If she would like her partner to put in her diaphragm, it could be fun, or at least funny. These can be slippery, and it is not difficult to imagine the diaphragm flying across the room if care isn't taken to hold it firmly during application.

Start with the woman lying down on her back, with legs separated and slightly bent. Her partner should fill the diaphragm with spermicidal jelly, rubbing the jelly over the sides as well. The woman should then direct her partner to squeeze the diaphragm's sides together (this is where he might find himself with a projectile missile) and slowly insert it into the vagina, pressing slightly downward so that it ends up under the pubic bone. She will say whether or not it is inserted correctly. If not, take it out and try again. This could be very sexy if done right, or it can add a certain amount of humor to your lovemaking if done ineptly.

Putting on a condom is a bit of an art, too. The male should lie on his back and tell his partner how to place the condom on the head of the penis and slowly roll it down until it covers the full shaft. This can be done very slowly and seductively, while touching the scrotum and nibbling on his nipples.

> *I placed the condom on the tip of his penis in the usual way and then unrolled it by drawing the penis into my mouth and pushing the rolled edge all the way down with my lips. This works best with the flavored lubricated variety.*

If the female partner is not very wet naturally, supplement with a great lubricant. In chapter 2 we recommended Astroglide if you are using a latex condom or Albolene cream if you are not. Some people like products made with aloe—which also makes the genitals feel smooth and silky. Applying lubrication can be a sexy part of foreplay, so you may want to use it even if the woman is naturally very moist. Each should put a little bit on the other partner, gently touching different parts of the genitalia until each person is slick and aroused. A slow, sensual approach changes an ordinary act into an erotic one.

> *I really enjoyed your instructions for how my husband should use a lubricant on me. I used to feel like a piece of bread being slathered with butter. This approach was a real turn-on.*

Beyond the Missionary Position

Woman on Top

We recommend a woman-on-top position as a starting point. After all, it *is* Sadie Hawkins Day, and in this position the woman has greater control over the depth of penetration and pace of thrusting. There are several variations on this theme :

BASIC—He's lying down and she's on top, facing him. She can be on her knees with forearms extended. This allows less depth of penetration but is easier to sustain for a longer time.

INTERMEDIATE—Partners are on a chair and she is sitting on his lap, facing him. Penetration is deep, but thrusting is limited because you are so close. Done slowly, this can be a very sensual position.

ADVANCED—He's lying on his back. She can squat over him, balance on her feet, and have a lot of leverage lowering herself down on him. (She needs good balance and strength to do this for any length of time. It can also be tricky if the bed is not very firm, so this might be better done on the floor.)

In these positions, the partners are face-to-face. You can look deeply into each other's eyes and see each other's expressions. Maintaining eye contact can be tremendously intimate and exciting. Both partners can lean over and kiss each other. The man can touch the woman's clitoris, her breasts and nipples, or grip her buttocks firmly. The woman can touch and gently pinch the man's nipples and she can reach down and guide his penis into her, then reach back, touching the scrotum from time to time. She can also easily reach for more lubricant if she needs it. Also, these positions aid in delaying the man's orgasm.

We suggest a lot of clitoral touching, either by the male, the woman touching herself, or both. Let the woman control penetration and pace; she should keep shifting angles to see which one feels the best to her and her partner. Try moving the shaft of the penis against the pubic bone, then as far away from it as possible. Touch the clitoris in long strokes or in short ones. Touch the labia gently as they touch the penis shaft. Women should stroke the penis as it goes in and out, occasionally reaching back to stroke the testicles and inner thighs. See how many different sensations can be experienced, and make sure the other person knows what really feels good to you, what you would like repeated or sustained—or remembered when you return to lovemaking in everyday life.

Spoon Position

This position is a very cuddly way of making love. There is a lot of close contact for the bodies, and it is easy to do for a long time. The woman's back is pressed against the man's front and he is entering from the rear.

Although the couple cannot see each other unless the man lifts his head and leans over the woman, nor can the woman easily touch the man, there is a lot of full body contact with this position. The woman can relax and just be made love to. The man's hands are free to caress the woman's breasts and genitals, and the woman's hands are free for her to touch her clitoris or labia. The woman can control depth of penetration. This is a 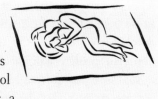 good position for women who prefer shallow penetration. And finally, this position is not too physically taxing and the man, especially, doesn't have to worry about getting tired out.

Rear Entry

We tried them all, but our favorite is the rear entry with my wife's back really arched. It allows the penis to penetrate deeper.

This is a position that men seem to like a lot. There are three main variations:

BASIC—The woman is on her stomach, arms outstretched, palms down, or she is propped up on her elbows. A pillow can be placed under her pelvis to raise her slightly. This position is easy for her if she can find a comfortable position. The man is holding his weight by outstretching his arms, his hands on each side of her hips, his legs between her legs and outstretched behind him.

INTERMEDIATE—The woman is on her knees, either with straight arms or on her elbows. The straight arms require more strength. The man is on his knees and his hands are either on his partner's back or, for maximum penetration, on her buttocks. In this latter position, he is straight-backed, moving his hips straight into her.

EXOTIC—The man is seated on a chair, and the woman sits on him, facing away from him. She has a lot of control over penetration; he doesn't have to work very hard.

For Sadie Hawkins Day, this position may not be the one that gives the woman a sense of control. The woman doesn't have much freedom of movement, but some women enjoy not having to reciprocate for a while. If the man penetrates deeply, the woman has very little ability to subtly determine the degree of penetration or pace.

However, men especially find this position erotic, because it allows them to set the pace of their thrusts. Some women occasionally like giving this sense of control to their partner. Some men love what, for them, is optimally deep penetration.

Many men find looking at their partner's buttocks and watching the penis move in and out to be extremely erotic.

Being able to see one's self in a mirror is a bonus. The man can reach around and easily stroke the clitoris and vulva. This is very exciting when combined with holding the buttocks and thrusting.

While this position is highly stimulating to many men, it also gives them some control against rapid ejaculation because they can easily withdraw when they get close to orgasm.

Face-to-Face, Side by Side

We like face-to-face, side by side. It is the most intimate to us because we have our hands and arms free to hold each other.

In this position the man and woman face each other, looking into each other's eyes, and have almost full body contact. The woman puts her leg over the man's hip, allowing him to enter her at an angle. Her arm is around his shoulder, while one of the man's arms is stretched out under his head or is helping to support his body. The other arm is free, and the hand can touch her breasts or reach down and touch her genital area.

While the woman has only a little maneuvering room and might find holding her position over him tiring, this one is not physically taxing. Because the couple is face-to-face, they can maintain more frequent eye contact, and kiss easily and often during lovemaking. This position allows medium penetration, more than in the spoon position but not as much as woman above or man behind. It allows a lot of contact with the labia and the clitoris, and because it is a more unusual position, it might be stimulating just because it allows penetration in a new angle.

The woman can stroke the man's face, touch his chest, and move away a little bit and touch his penis as it glides in and out. She has some control over depth of penetration, and there is mutual control over the pace of thrusting.

The Climax

After you have tried as many of these positions as you desire and you are very excited, you can choose to do one of two things: climax in a new position (or a less familiar one), or have your orgasm in the tried-and-true way, just to make sure you get exactly what you want.

Interlude: Time-Out After Sex

After you have had a really terrific orgasm, we want you to take it easy. A couple cannot live by sex alone. Part of any intimate vacation is varying the main event with other pleasures. We recommend an all-afternoon break. Almost anything you enjoy doing together is fine. However, we strongly suggest not choosing a competitive activity, such as tennis, even if you normally enjoy playing against each other. We don't want a bad game to spoil anyone's mood. (You don't want to engage in a very strenuous activity. Keep your outings brief and leisurely.)

- Shop together for fun (e.g., go antique or bargain hunting, but look for interesting rather than functional items).
- Take in an upbeat funny or romantic movie.
- Relax in your own garden or wander in some public gardens.
- Have lunch at a wonderful café or view restaurant.
- Go for an easy hike and a picnic (bring along books to read to each other or read individually in each other's company).
- Explore a new area together.
- Visit a museum together or stroll through a few art galleries.
- Rest by the hotel's pool or Jacuzzi (or a coed facility at a local health club).
- Take a drive in the country if you can avoid stress-inducing superhighways.
- Go horseback riding.
- Go ice-skating or in-line skating.

We took our afternoon break touring the chocolate factory in Las Vegas—chocolate is one of our favorite aphrodisiacs. We came home and took a nap in each other's arms.

LATE AFTERNOON: TAKE IT EASY

We combined our afternoon break and rest time by napping cuddled in a blanket in the sun at the beach.

Depending on the time of day and your own preferences, you might save time at the end of the day for a short nap (or you could take the whole afternoon, skipping all our suggestions, and take a long nap). In fact, if you haven't used the Happy Massager® earlier, this might be the perfect time to use it. If you wish, take a nap and wake each other up with five to ten minutes of back and leg massages. Naps are not only physically restorative, but quieting your minds together creates more intimacy. In any case, take some time to relax before getting ready for dinner.

5

Saturday Evening

I surprised him by bringing new lingerie and a feather boa to wear with a push-up bra and high heels to do a striptease. He surprised me by bringing our camcorder and set it up to project my striptease onto the TV screen. I loved watching myself. It was a great turn-on for both of us.

YOU'VE HAD YOUR DAY OUT, AND MAYBE A nap, too. We hope you feel refreshed and ready for dinner. We suggest a little predinner verbal foreplay.

HORS D'OEUVRES: VERBAL FOREPLAY BEFORE DINNER

EXERCISE 1: *Exchange Wish List and Sex Checks (Highly Recommended)*
Over a relaxing drink, talk about plans for this evening and Sunday. What would you like to do that you haven't

done yet? What would your partner like to try? Is there anything that you would like to repeat? Each person makes a wish list. This is also a good time to exchange the Sex Checks discussed in chapter 2. You could also make your *own* wish list by creating a personalized IOU and exchanging as many as you like now. You can have some fun by giving your partner a signed blank IOU as a playful open-ended invitation. Your partner gets a fantasy fulfilled, while you get the delight of a spontaneous surprise. You can then decide whether you want to grant the wish or redeem a check or IOU tonight or tomorrow, or sometime after the weekend, as a way to carry over new ideas into real life.

Personal Fantasy

I.O.U.

I promise you _____

_____

_____

_____

_____

EXERCISE 2: *Swapping Fantasies*

What are some of the things that you think about when you fantasize? (You don't really want to upset your partner by naming other people or admitting you sometimes pretend your partner is someone else while making love.) Tell your partner why the imagery you describe is so arousing for you. Describe which images you want to keep only as fantasy and which ones you might want to act out a little—or a lot.

This exercise can be a bit dangerous, because there are some fantasies that shouldn't be revealed. However, the better you know and understand each other—and the more nonjudgmental you and your partner are—the more risks you can take. But sharing fantasies can be very arousing, and the trust that such exchanges demonstrates helps forge an increased sense of intimacy.

He told me that he pictured me going down on him while we're driving on an empty desert highway. I said someday I'd love to have sex in a hotel Jacuzzi late at night, knowing that other guests might be watching from their windows.

I told him that I frequently fantasized that we're making love outdoors. When we got back from dinner, we had sex on a blanket on the bathroom floor with the heat lamp and pretended that we were outside in the hot sun.

DINNER: VERBAL FOREPLAY AND MORE . . .

We recommend going out tonight. Being in one place too long may become claustrophobic. Besides, going out to dinner encourages you to dress attractively and behave intimately and seductively. If you choose to stay at home, this is a good time for a joint cooking project.

At this dinner, celebrate your closeness. Design your evening in one of two ways: You can make the evening nonsexual but romantic, or you can make it sexual and playful. No matter which option you choose, this evening is a good time to exchange great relationship stories and enjoy being together. You might want to recount the most romantic moments you've shared. Take turns describing your favorite memories, or recollect the best sex you've ever had together and why it was so good. Describe the experience in as much detail as you can from the first to last touch.

OPTION: *A Dinner Game—*
Fantasy Role-Playing

Role-playing allows both of you to explore different parts of your imaginations that you wouldn't normally play out in real life. So try playacting as someone else. The biggest challenge is to keep yourself from feeling stupid or "breaking out of character." Still, if you can agree that you are in this "play" together, this exercise can be sexier than you might at first imagine. It's like having an affair without violating promises of monogamy.

In the most satisfying role-playing, your character's words and actions should come forth without reservation. If you start the role-playing in a public place, you are more likely to carry through with the scenario. (Also, having an audience for your bold flirtation with a "total stranger" can be a terrific turn-on.) In private, try to include positions and sex acts that the characters you are playing would want but that you might be reluctant to try as "yourselves." Keep in mind that whatever your partner does, this is a game. It's acting—like in the movies—and you're merely trying on another person's reality for a little while. If you have never done this before, pick a scenario that seems emotionally comfortable. And if you crack up laughing a few times, great; but then pull yourself together and continue. The idea is to be playful, titillating, and most of all, to have fun. Here are a few scenarios you might enjoy:

THE SEDUCTION. You are meeting each other for the first time. Walk separately into a restaurant for dinner and sit down at different tables. Pretend that you are strangers who start eyeing each other. One of you can walk over and introduce yourself. Or ask the waiter/waitress to pass the other person a note saying how attractive you find him or her. The interaction with your server helps keep you in character. The person who receives the note can either motion the sender to come over or walk to the sender's table, say "hello," and sit down. Begin to flirt with each other. You can imagine that this is the beginning of a great love affair, or just a prelude to one stolen afternoon of pure lust.

I always thought my fiancé was a tad reticent, but he had a surprise in store for me. He walked away to the bar for our drinks and came back someone else! He began role-playing and all of a sudden there was this lovely man trying to pick me up. We were still ourselves, but we were strangers. He offered to buy me a drink and asked permission to join me. We flirted and laughed and made small talk for a couple of hours. We discovered the freedom to talk about things the way you do to someone you may never see again. He told me things about "his relationship" that he had never said before. What delicious revelations. He actually expressed feelings I suspected were inside of him but were kept hidden for years.

We pretended we just met and had instant chemistry. We went back to "his place." Somewhere in the middle of the great sex, we became ourselves again and continued the lovemaking with lovely familiarity.

SEX FOR SALE. Make believe one of you is "for hire." He could be an elegant escort, or she a high-priced, exclusive call girl. He could be a young man having his first sexual experience with a mature "woman of the world." Or it's her first time, so she picked a Don Juan to introduce her to the mysteries of sex. This could be a very titillating scenario to play out at home or on the town.

I couldn't believe how much he looked like an "escort." He came to the door in an elegant Italian suit. The hottest part was dancing; he had a hard-on, his body never left mine, and he kept asking me what I wanted and then told me how he could give it to me.

LIVES OF THE RICH AND FAMOUS. One of you can pretend to be a famous actor, rock star, athlete, or model whom you both find sexy; the other can be the "admirer" who is selected for "quick" intimacy. You come up to him or her in a restaurant for an autograph. The "star" shows immediate and unmistakable interest in you. Or both of you can be famous and you are trying to explore your attraction while avoiding the prying eyes and cameras of your fans and paparazzi. You want to be intimate, but of course everyone is watching. Eventually, you separately sneak back to your private hideaway.

After Dinner: Relaxing and Struggling

We have some romantic videos that are meaningful to us. Mostly they are sunsets and seascapes (some we have taped ourselves and some from pre-bought videos). They are calm and soothing.

We don't want you to feel as if you have embarked on an exhausting sexual marathon. Unless you have turned each other on so much that you want more, more, more, you might want to return to your bedroom or hotel room and just cuddle and be close tonight. Some road-testers had the energy and desire to go out after dinner, and chose activities consistent with the weekend theme of trying things that are a bit out of the ordinary.

My husband surprised me by taking me to a strip club! I'd never been to one before. He brought twenty dollars in singles to tip the dancers, then invited a beautiful young woman to join us at our table, which was arousing for both of us. We stayed for about an hour and enjoyed watching the women be seductive, and I picked up some stripping tips to use later that night.

If you don't want another sexual exercise, but you do want some more stimulation before going to sleep, we have a couple of suggestions:

OPTION: *Enjoy a Rented Movie Together in the Comfort of Bed*

Pick a light romantic comedy or drama you've enjoyed in the past but haven't seen in years. Add a trip to a video store to your afternoon outing plans and bring a videotape back to enjoy at home or at the hotel (if your room is equipped with a VCR).

If you would like to watch a sexy but not X-rated video, here are some titles from *Playboy*'s recently published list of films that feature their favorite "searing movie scenes":

☆ *Body Heat*

☆ *The Postman Always Rings Twice*

☆ *Don't Look Now*

☆ *Risky Business*

☆ *sex, lies and videotape*

☆ *Breathless*

☆ *The Big Easy*

☆ *Atlantic City*   ☆ *The Lover*
☆ *The Last Seduction*   ☆ *White Palace*
☆ *Sea of Love*   ☆ *The Hunger*
☆ *Look Twice*   ☆ *9½ Weeks*
☆ *The Unbearable*
   Lightness of Being

Here are a few other romantic video suggestions provided by our road-test couples and *Glamour* magazine readers:

☆ *Top Gun*   ☆ *Bull Durham*
☆ *The English Patient*   ☆ *The Bodyguard*
☆ *Jerry Maguire*   ☆ *Blue Sky*
☆ *Don Juan de Marco*   ☆ *Sleepless in Seattle*
☆ *When Harry Met Sally*   ☆ *Henry and June*
☆ *True Romance*   ☆ *Desert Hearts*
☆ *Belle de Jour*   ☆ *An Officer and a*
                                                Gentleman

OPTION: *A Candlelit Bath*
Place candles around the bathtub before dinner, so your only postdinner tasks are turning on the tap and lighting a match. The more candles, the better. We also recommend using your bubble bath, bath salts, or aromatic oils. Just settle into each other's arms and relax; if sex starts all over again, so be it, but it's not the point.

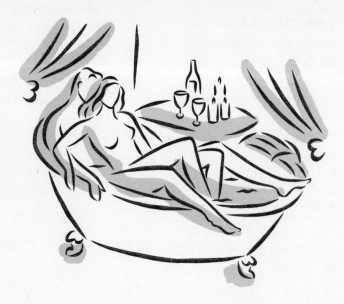

We combined our candlelit bath with dinner. We ate pad Thai-noodles right from the take-out container with chopsticks in a nice, cozy candlelit tub. It was very decadent and indulgent!

OPTION: *Full-Body Massages*

We gave each other full-body massages and did food play. He dripped honey down my body, saying, "Not that you need to be any sweeter . . ."

To begin, partners can sit at opposite ends of a sofa, each with his or her foot in the other's lap. Massage each other's foot, experimenting with strokes and pressure, then tell each other how the rubbing and pressure points feel to you. Wipe off excess oil so your feet won't be slippery.

Debra D'Amato, our Beverly Hills masseuse friend, offers a few simple ground rules: Give feedback; it's okay to moan, ooh and aah, or say "ouch." Let your partner know what feels good and what doesn't.

When you are ready to move to the next stage, one partner finds a comfortable place to lie facedown, while the other warms his or her hands and prepares to give a massage. Massage the back and shoulders; that's where most people hold the majority of their tension. Once that area is relaxed, move down to the buttocks and legs. After the person turns over, gently massage the neck and head, then work all the way down the front of the body to the feet. Remember, this massage is for pleasure, not for sexual arousal. Some people like their stomach massaged and others don't, so ask. That's a sensitive body part, so go easy and gentle. Another tip from D'Amato: Warm the oil in

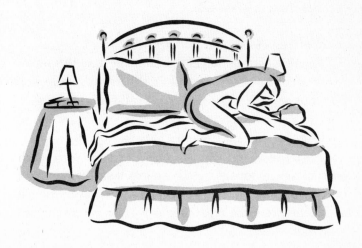

your hands, then follow the grain of the muscle and work *toward* the heart.

For those who aren't accustomed to exchanging massages, start with a 10- to 15-minute massage, then switch roles—any longer and you risk losing out because your partner might fall asleep. Those accustomed to giving and getting massage know what they like and can take as long as they like. D'Amato's last tip: Close your eyes and just let your hands feel your partner's body get lost in the process. Giving *can* be as wonderful as receiving.

> We purchased scented oil that smelled like passion fruit and massaged each other with it. We alternated with our hands and "Mr. Happy" in order to give each other a longer massage. It felt good to give that much.

> We bought a cheap shower curtain and put it on the floor. We drizzled about a half a cup of vegetable oil and one half cup of warm water over it. We started with back rubs and slipped and slided into sex.

Putting More Play in Your Passion

Even though you might not normally have this much sex in a day, some of you will find that you get aroused from the sex talk. If the evening is still young, you might want to give more pleasure to each other and try one of the following optional exercises tonight.

For those of you who are ready for more out-of-the-ordinary sex, Saturday night is an excellent time to make things really last—to introduce play as well as passion—and to try not to be orgasm-driven. Here are a smorgasbord of possibilities—some are rated exotic for the really adventurous.

OPTION: *Body Exploration*

This is a shortened version of the pleasuring exercise from Friday night. You can do it again if you liked it, or for the first time if you didn't indulge on Friday night. The woman touches the man first, then he follows and does everything she did to him, plus thinks of places that she missed. Take turns touching each other for a long time before intercourse is "allowed."

OPTION: *Adult (X-rated) Video*

Watching a video is a good idea when one or both partners are not yet in an erotic mood but want to be. Those who have never opted for this form of arousal may use this special weekend as an opportunity to try it. See "Recommended Adult Videos" at the end of this book for some popular titles. Of course, using adult videos as a sex aid is old hat to some couples, and this provides an opportunity to do what they know they like. These couples might see this as a time to order or rent something that seems a bit far out.

> *My husband and I have been married for 15 years and I thought I knew him. I thought he would never agree to watch an X-rated movie and if he did, he'd be grossed out. I was shocked when he consented but even more surprised at how quickly he got excited. We watched about five minutes of the movie and then he was all over me—very, very hot. I'm sure we'll try this again.*

Angela Cohen, coauthor of *The Wild Woman's Guide to Erotic Videos,* recommends good, offbeat films such as *Cafe Flesh* (a futuristic cult film), *Dracula Exotic* (the classic story, retold), or *The Hottest Bid* (men being auctioned at a fund-raiser).

Erotic-film director Lizzie Borden suggests that people who have difficulty expressing what they want in words or giving directions use the video to show their partner what they want or like by replaying specific scenes. Like the Sex Checks, the video can provide a way for couples to communicate without talking as they watch and respond to the film together. Or you can leave it on for its sounds of sex as background noise while you make love. If you're feeling in the mood, pretend the cameras are focused on you and your partner, and try to be sexier or naughtier than the porn stars.

> *We enjoyed watching a porno movie together because it seemed like we were having sex in the same room as those characters in the film.*

OPTION: *Private Role-Playing Games*

If you didn't engage in role-playing during dinner, you might want to play out a scenario now. Some fantasies are best acted out in private. If you do your own scene, or one suggested below, try to include sex acts or positions that your characters would want but that you would be reluctant to try in real life.

THE WEDDING NIGHT. Replay your own wedding night as you would have liked it to be, if you knew then what you know now. If it was perfect, take pleasure in reenacting the event. Set the stage. Are you at a beach in Fiji? What do you each look like? Or imagine you are both virgins. What will you teach each other? (Or, if you like, pretend one of you is the expert who will provide the perfect sexual and romantic initiation.)

THE LOVE SLAVE. You played poker—and lost. You bet everything on the last hand. At stake was your freedom, for one act of sexual pleasuring. And now you have to pay. You have to do *everything* the victor demands. The victor—secretly in love with the vanquished—makes sexual demands but ultimately wants the slave to end up craving more.

But these are just a few of our suggestions. Here are some sexy scenarios our road-testers came up with:

> We tried two. In the afternoon, we drove around the countryside. I played the role of a chauffeur; she was a French mistress. We never stepped out of those roles the entire afternoon. It was a gas! Sunday, my wife donned our daughter's old cheerleading outfit and we went from there.

> My husband was a pirate and I was a saucy lass posing as a cabin boy to get passage to Barbados (escaping a life of indentured servitude, of course). The pirate feels a strange attraction to the cabin boy (who tries hard to hide her gender!) and is quite relieved to find out she's a woman.

OPTION: *Body Painting*

This can be a lot of fun. Many couples find it erotic to draw on each other's body. If this appeals to you, we hope

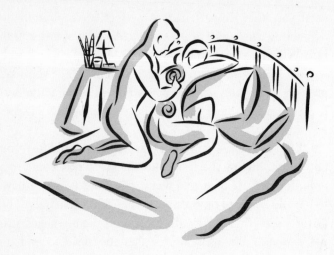

you planned ahead and bought the nontoxic body paints described in chapter 3. You may want to do this in the bathtub or shower, or in the bedroom with your old sheets, towels, or with a plastic paint tarp on the bed or floor. Take turns decorating each other's chest, breasts, back, buttocks, and genital area. Challenge yourself to integrate a specific body part into the scenery. The more imagination you use, the more fun it is. Plus, the brush strokes and wet paint feel quite sensuous on bare skin.

When you have finished your handiwork, you might want to think about photographing each other with a Polaroid camera (of course, if you're at all worried about photos being discovered, we recommend destroying them before the end of the weekend). Washing each other off should be a slow, seductive experience. It might lead to sex in the bathtub or shower—which is the next option of the evening.

Take your own sheets if you go to a hotel. We trashed a set of sheets with chocolate and peanut butter and had to change them. I would have been mortified if this happened to the hotel's linens.

OPTION: *Sex Under Water*

Albolene is way too slippery for regular sex, but we thought it was great for water sex.

If you have sex in the bathtub, enjoy the feeling of the waves around your body and try not to flood the place! Also, take care to bring your lubricant with you, because the water will dry out a woman's vaginal passage and can make intercourse painful. You don't want to have to end the weekend early because of soreness.

Or you might want to experiment with sex standing up in the shower. However, depending on your relative heights, lovemaking in the shower may be easier or more difficult than in the bath. Remember, both showers and tubs can be slippery. Don't let passion send you to the emergency room. That stated, making love with water streaming down your back in a hot steamy room can be both sensual and astoundingly erotic. Again, make sure you use a lot of lubricant in the shower, because the water may make penetration and thrusting more difficult.

OPTION: *Hot and Cold Oral Sex*

This is an exciting variation on the theme of prolonging your sexual experiences. Slowly lick, suck, and gently create a rhythm. Ask your partner to let you know what feels best. Tell your partner what feels good. What felt good on Friday night is not necessarily what your partner wants now. After you have your partner very aroused, prepare to give (and receive) a real treat. Get some ice (small crescent-shaped cubes are best) and put it by the bedside. Put a small cube in your mouth for a few seconds, then remove it. Put your mouth on your partner's genitals quickly, while your mouth is still cold; your natural body temperature will make your mouth warm again, and your partner should love the alternating warm and cold feeling.

If you want to be truly exotic, bring a cup of hot tea to bed and swill some in your mouth before swallowing. Alternating ice and hot tea gives your partner the thrill of going from cold to hot and back again. You can become adept at holding the ice cube in your cheek and moving it to your lips, holding it there, then teasing the entire genital area. All of these variations on using hot and cold during oral sex can provide intense pleasure and unforgettable orgasm.

We decided to do this exercise blindfolded so each sensation would be a surprise.

OPTION: *Tantric Sex*

Gazing into her eyes and feeling the rhythm of our breathing took me beyond our bodies to a profound level of love.

Tantric sex is the ancient sacred Hindu art of making love. We cannot do justice to this deep, intricate philosophy here, but the basic premise is to use focused breathing as a way to unify yourself mentally, physically, and spiritually. By sharing tantric exercises with a partner, couples can reach a powerful emotional connection. Western culture typically separates sexuality from spirituality, and tantric exercises are a way to integrate them in a way that leads to a higher order of intimacy, sensuality, and orgasmic capacity.

You can have a great time exploring these exotic options even as a novice. Typically, couples face each other and synchronize their breathing. This exercise is a good way to slow down the pace of lovemaking and tune in to your partner. Try this position: Sitting naked, the male sits on the floor and the female sits on top of him, facing him with her legs over his, curling them around his waist for support; his legs can either be extended or curled around her buttocks. Each person places his or her right hand over the partner's heart. Maintaining eye contact, breathe slowly and deeply together for at least five minutes. (You can also do this standing face-to-face, or standing or lying in the spoon positions, chest-to-back.)

Breathing can also be used to intensify orgasm: About halfway into your climax, try drawing in your breath as slowly as possible; the intensity of your sensations will build for as long as you can sustain the inhalation. Then, when you have to exhale, let the air out in a noisy whoosh. Some tantric practitioners claim the more noise you make, the better your orgasm will feel. If you get really good at this, the orgasm can be extended with three or four additional exhalations!

If these exercises entice you to know more about tantric sex, you'll find much more detailed explanations in books like *Tantra: The Art of Conscious Living* by Charles and Caroline Muir. Couples who incorporate tantra can enter a sexual meditation that has blissful results.

OPTION SEVEN: *Extending Your Orgasms*

The goal of this exercise is to have mental control over your body in order to intensify sensation. Delaying orgasm as long as possible may well give you one of the most intense climaxes you have ever had. You probably won't get this right the first time you try, but the attempt will be fun.

Men: You will practice a form of discipline that trains you to get right up to the point of ejaculation and then stop, so that you learn to know when to save yourself for more stimulation. Sex therapists recommend withdrawal at the edge of ejaculation and the practice of the "squeeze technique"—which involves firmly squeezing the underside of the penis, where the head meets the shaft. A four-second squeeze to this part of the penis greatly diminishes the urge to ejaculate. Don't get upset if you misjudge how close you are; enjoy your orgasm and consider practicing this technique another time. If you are successful with this, you will probably feel a difference when you finally allow yourself to climax.

If you want to move on to the exotic level of this exercise, which includes learning to have multiple orgasms by separating orgasm from ejaculation, read *The Multi-Orgasmic Man* by Mantak Chia and Douglas Abrams Arava. Combining Western scientific knowledge with ancient Chinese sexual wisdom, the authors try to teach men how to have several whole-body orgasms without losing their erection, saving ejaculation until the final climax.

Women: Allow your partner to bring you to the brink

but stopping short of orgasm. This can be done during either intercourse, petting, or oral sex. Give your partner a signal about how long you are really willing to hold off your climax. Try not to hurry your climax or make it happen. Let it overtake you. When you are ready to have the world's most splendid orgasm, make sure you let your partner know so it doesn't accidentally get derailed by a change in tempo or withdrawal of stimulation. Communicate in a sexy whisper or shout "Don't stop," or "I'm ready to come."

Remember, the point is to stay on the edge of orgasm, as close as you can, for as long as you can. Of course, women are multiorgasmic more frequently than men. Women may wish to come quickly, but let your partner know that on this special night you want seconds, thirds, or more!

THE NIGHT ENDS

We suspect that you're probably ready for a deep sleep. Make sure you're well rested for the last day of your weekend of great sex.

Usually we move to our own sides of the bed to get a good night's rest, but Saturday we fell asleep in each other's arms. Being that close generated a warm glow that lasted all day Sunday.

6

Sunday Morning

My wife woke me up and fed me from a plate of warmed nectarine slices and morsels of chocolate cake with chocolate frosting that had all been moistened with cream. After indulging in this decadence, we naturally fell into deep kisses and caresses. My favorite love songs played softly in the background.

SUNDAY MORNINGS ARE THE TIMES TO BE lazy. So sleep in. Breakfast in bed is always a treat. Use room service, or if cooking is your idea of fun, cook something special together, or pamper your partner a little. If you prefer, go out to a little café and bring back warm muffins and gourmet coffee. Just enjoy the moment.

Shower together or apart before trying the morning exercises. But don't make love in the shower. We have some other playful options for you to try this morning.

My husband heated my towel in the dryer and presented it to me when I stepped out of the shower. He wanted to make the shower extra special, and he did.

Now that your Sunday morning is off to a nice, slow start, you might be ready to choose your last sexy exercises for the weekend.

EXERCISE 1: *Sex Toys*

Even in the quiet early-morning hours, you may prefer something with bells, whistles, and batteries. For those of you who already know you like sex toys, try a new one. Or, if you bought your first sex toy as part of your preparation for your Great Sex Weekend, you and your partner will probably be comfortable and confident enough now to experiment.

I bought my girlfriend a Hitachi Magic Wand vibrator with a G-Spot attachment as a surprise gift. First I gave her a full-body massage. Then we put on the G-Spot attachment up her bottom and we had sex. I could feel the vibrations—it was great! Later we laid it under her and I was in her, and again it was terrific. This was a first for both of us.

My boyfriend loved watching me reach multiple orgasms with my vibrator, because they are so intense. I never used one before, and it has really opened new doors to my sexuality.

If, when you were planning this weekend, you thought toys held no appeal for you or your partner, but by Sunday morning you've changed your mind, it may not be too late. The local sex boutique may be open on Sunday. Go pick out something together. Pick out something more outrageous than you would ordinarily select.

If there are no such boutiques in your area, you're still in luck. Regular stores have useful items. Well-stocked drugstores carry an array of electric massagers, some with a variety of attachments. The Hitachi Magic Wand, our favorite, can be used as a vibrator. Silk scarves from department stores make perfect blindfolds. Grocery stores have whipped cream, puddings, and other foodstuffs that you can incorporate into your love play.

EXERCISE 2: *Talking Sexy*

We think talking sexy can be incorporated into any of the exercises in this book. Once cultivated, this skill can help keep your sex life very lively indeed. You can get exactly what you want in bed, but *only* if you feel comfortable asking for it, and *only* if your partner feels comfortable about being told what to do.

We usually assume our partner can intuit our feelings so they don't have to be expressed. Yet few of us are mind readers. And even if we think we know how our partner feels, it's still a turn-on to *hear* the words. By simply stating aloud what is going on and how it makes you feel, you give your partner extreme pleasure and a sense of security. And this is very arousing.

> *My usually quiet lover turned into a very vocal man, describing in great detail what he was doing, what he was going to do, and then doing it. The sex talk was incredibly exciting and scintillating. We had the best sex ever. Slowly, deliberately, he narrated with a passion that was beyond belief.*

Sentiments That You Might Want to Communicate to Your Partner

WOMEN

☆ compliments about his body or facial features

☆ how his hands feel on your body

☆ how you love the way his penis looks, how hard it is

☆ how much you are turned on when he enters or "fills" you

☆ how he feels inside you

☆ how it feels when he starts going fast/slow/gentle/hard

☆ how much you love him

MEN

☆ how her skin feels

☆ how her breasts feel

☆ how great it feels to grasp her to you

☆ what you are thinking about when you first enter her

☆ how she feels to you when you're inside her

☆ how much you love her

We use sexier language while we're making love now. Having said those words once made it easier to use them again.

The Chinese Menu Game

In her book *Talk Sexy to the One You Love (and Drive Each Other Wild in Bed)*, which we recommend to readers who want to go explore more verbal exercises, Barbara

Keesling suggests writing out, then whispering, speaking aloud—even shouting—the words that complete these sentences: "I want to (<u>verb</u>) your (<u>noun</u>)." and "I want you to (<u>verb</u>) my (<u>noun</u>)."

We've taken Keesling's exercise a little further by adding adjectives and adverbs, and suggest the following choices to spur you on. By all means, add your own words

ADVERBS	VERBS	ADJECTIVES	NOUNS
slowly	caress	beautiful	cock/penis
gently	nibble	sexy	balls
fast	suck	virile	breasts/tits
hard	tickle	hard	tummy
teasingly	fuck	sleek	bottom/butt/
lightly	spank	taut	ass
mercilessly	pull/tug	round	thighs
lovingly	bite	strong	shoulders
passionately	tease	soft	feet/toes
sensuously	lick	hairy/hairless	clitoris
carefully	flick your	(color: pink,	G-spot
wildly	tongue	red)	fingers
wickedly	play with	long	nipples
firmly	undress	juicy, wet	chest
creatively	kiss	big	cunt/pussy/
powerfully	eat	delicious	vagina
calmly	touch	luscious	lips
	taste	lubricated	neck/throat
			ears
			eyelids

and phrases to the choices offered. Use them to complete these two sentences:

I want to (<u>adverb</u>) (<u>verb</u>) your (<u>adjective</u>) (<u>noun</u>).
I want you to (<u>adverb</u>) (<u>verb</u>) my (<u>adjective</u>) (<u>noun</u>).

Before lovemaking gets so passionate that the exercise is over, take one or more turns telling your partner something you want to do or asking for something you want. Hopefully, you'll grant each other's wishes but stay within everyone's comfort zone. Even if *you* don't want to try something, it's important to know your partner's sexual desires. If you are not ready to try a specific act at this time, you might consider visualizing your partner's desires during lovemaking or during your own masturbation after the weekend ends. Perhaps by your next sexy getaway, you'll be ready to grant your partner's wish.

We loved talking dirty to each other. We've never done it before, and we found it quite arousing.

Last Sex of the Weekend

The exercises you choose should lead to an exciting, open sexual experience. Keep communicating. Whisper, talk, grunt, moan. Try something new, or something old but favored. Just keep sharing your thoughts and feelings during this last encounter before you get ready for lunch and the transition back to the real world. Seize this last opportunity of your sexy getaway to really open up to each other.

7

Sunday Afternoon: Perfect Endings

Her note read: "Remembering your sweetly scented skin, gentle coaxing hands, and tender murmurings of encouragement. . . ."

THE TRANSITION FROM THE WEEKEND BACK to reality is as important as any other part of your getaway experience. Make this as gradual and unhurried as your best lovemaking. We recommend that you share your feelings about the weekend while they are fresh and you are feeling close and secure.

It should be lunchtime about now. If you've stayed home, it might be a good time to leave the house and go to a restaurant. Before you leave, put away the candles and the sex toys, put the stereo or VCR back in the family room—that is, do whatever it takes to get the house back to normal. (The Happy Massager® is not a sex toy; it's just a wonderful tool to help each other feel better. You can leave it by the bed and use it on yourself, your partner, or your kids. They'll love it, too.)

If you're in a hotel, check out, but don't take off for home just yet. Take time for one last meal somewhere calm and pleasant. Enjoy a leisurely lunch, but after the meal, we suggest that each person take the time to write a love letter to the other—maybe just a few short paragraphs—recollecting the best parts of the weekend and closing with some personal thoughts about your relationship and your feelings for your partner. Write down those notions that you rarely express, or comment on the wonderful little things that your partner does for you. Include a few private thoughts that you've never shared before. You want to touch your partner's heart. Later this evening, right before you go to bed, exchange your notes as the perfect ending for your weekend together.

> *I'm sorry that I don't tell you more often how attracted and in love I am with you. You are my man! You are my life!*

> *I feel so alive when we are totally immersed sharing ourselves with each other. I love you.*

> *He wrote, "Honey, I really didn't know how sexy you are capable of being until this weekend. I now look at you as my sex goddess."*

When you exchange the letters, spend some time talking about your feelings. This is a good time to plan for a future sex weekend. Get out your calendars and pick a date. It's important to plan your getaway and make it real by choosing an actual date. Perhaps you want to tie it into an upcoming vacation or a weekend when you know your children will be away from home.

> We wrote letters to each other. It made us realize how important our sex lives are to us. We each promised to make time for another romantic weekend soon.

We hope that real life will be even better now that you've had your first weekend getaway. Not every couple's weekend will live up to their expectations. Sometimes a workaholic just can't shake thinking or talking about the office. Or one partner enjoys the champagne a little too much, falls asleep early, and there goes the whole evening. Unpredictable things can happen. One road-test couple reported that the wife got food poisoning at a good restaurant; another reported that the baby-sitter canceled at the last minute. If the weekend needs to be rescheduled, don't give up.

Fortunately, other than a few minor mishaps, the Great Sex Weekend got rave reviews from the road-testers. Not everything in this program suits every couple, and some couples put together a program more tailored to their own style and tastes. This isn't the last word in sexy weekends. To the contrary, it's evident that all the elements of this weekend could be reconfigured. Like a good recipe, the basic ingredients are here and couples can pick and choose what they like, adding their own favorite activities—like flavorings and spices, so to speak. More important, this program should encourage couples to communicate better—to say those things that are thought but not spoken, and ask for those things that are wanted but never requested. Some couples who have been to-gether a long time have developed some telepathy about each other's needs, but many others get stuck in taking care of the details of everyday life and stop talking about their love, commitment, dreams, and desires.

After two kids and ten years of marriage, we'd slipped into a sexual rut. The book gave us an incentive to break our pattern. Now we're closer and more open to fun in bed than before.

The Great Sex Weekend is a way back to that kind of sharing. Sure, it is about sex and sensuality, but it is also about intimacy. And intimacy means opening up to each other, generously creating pleasure for each other, and re-membering to be lovers who are full of curiosity about how to please and know each other better. This book can help remind you that if you give each other full attention for even just a weekend, and create a playful, amorous atmosphere, your sexual and emotional relationship can be rejuvenated. Once you've done that, the next challenge is to not let the spirit and excitement of this weekend fade away. Now you have the tools to infuse the reality of your everyday lives with the pleasures and insights of these past two days.

I wish we could do this every weekend! (All week, too!) I wish I could always have all the time in the world to devote to my marriage, but unfortunately, the more mundane (and less important) parts of my life tend to take over. Our next getaway—on our anniversary—won't come soon enough!

8

Making Love in Everyday Life

We'd been living together for 11 years when we took our getaway weekend. About a week after we returned, she brought me coffee as I was stepping out of the shower. Without thinking, I asked her to do me the honor of marrying me. She said she'd have to think about it. A week later she said yes. I don't know what I would've done if she had turned me down.

E HOPE THIS TIME-OUT FOR SEX AND intimacy has encouraged you to feel really good about yourself and your relationship. This is a good time to think about your sex life and love life and what you gained from your weekend experience that you'd like to carry into everyday life.

Take an assessment of your usual lovemaking schedule. How often do you have sex (honestly)? There is no "right" answer. The frequency of sex for ALL couples diminishes significantly after the first year of a relationship and then decreases slowly over time. On average a couple may, depending in large part on age, have sex one to three times a week. In older relationships, a couple might be happy having sex as infrequently as once a month.

Review the last month before you started preparations for your sexy getaway. If the frequency was average for you, is that the amount of sex you or your partner want to have? If so, frequency is not a problem. However, if either of you feels that you make love too infrequently, discuss what would be a realistic amount of sex that would please you both. If you have different appetites, you might have to arrive at a compromise.

Do you often make love late at night, after 11 P.M., when you're both really too tired for a quality experience? When would be the perfect time? Sunday mornings? If you don't like sex in the morning, would you like to have sex on a weekend afternoon? If so, does that ever happen anymore? If you like having sex at night, is there some way you can both turn in early on nights when you're feeling amorous (or, at least, horny)? Should you turn off the TV earlier, or set the alarm ahead half an hour for more morning time together? Now that you've spent this luxurious time experimenting, how has it reminded you of the best ways to stage your sex life to maximize your energy and concentration?

Talk about feelings and events that get in the way of your lovemaking. Is it just that you are too tired during the week? Too wrapped up in errands or entertaining on the weekends? Should you make a pact never to talk about the children, or work, or money before you get into bed?

Does each of you initiate sex enough? Does your partner wish you initiated sex more often, or vice versa? Would you like Sadie Hawkins Day to occur at least once a month?

What was the most sexy or erotic way that you initiated sex this weekend? Did you begin having sex in a room other than the bedroom? Did the champagne put you in a sensual mood? What about seeing your partner in sexy underwear or lingerie? Did having breakfast in bed make you unusually playful? Did you enjoy trading massages on Saturday night? Should you take short weekend trips more often? In other words, what did you experience this weekend that could help you start hot—rather than mundane—sex?

Do you both set aside enough time for an occasional candlelit dinner at a restaurant or at home with the phone turned off? Many people think that such occasions should arise naturally and spontaneously. And sometimes they do. But they happen more often when couples are honest enough to admit that they need to take the time and make the effort to keep their romance vibrant.

While the glow of your Great Sex Weekend is still with you, take the opportunity to talk about the times when you feel more distant. How often do you feel out of touch with each other? This is a time for sharing. When both of you are feeling open and positive, it's much easier to talk about, and resolve, some of those long-standing issues: "It seems we can go several weeks without really connecting with each other. Does it seem like that to you, too?" Or, now is the time to initiate new rituals that will keep the spirit of your weekend alive—late-night chats (quality time) or walks together to enjoy quiet moments.

> *My husband is taking more time kissing me than he did before this weekend.*

> *We've done a lot more fantasy role-playing since the weekend. It's a great part of our sex life now.*

> *Beyond making time for each other and becoming more intimate, we have reestablished the lines of communication.*

> *After 11 years, we were like other couples who have lived together that long. We were way too busy and a little angry at the ways we took each other for granted. Instead of continuing to blame the other person, this book made us realize our problem was pretty common in these times. It gave us permission to treat ourselves. And we still make "dates" to be with each other, which we didn't do before.*

9

Your Next Getaway

I chose a beach resort for our first getaway, so my girlfriend picked a quiet mountain resort with very private cabins surrounded by redwoods for a completely different feel for our next one.

FUTURE WEEKEND TUNE-UPS

After all is said and done, you may decide that it's too difficult to restructure your sex life at home. It may be that the best you can do is plan another "time-out" to be lovers again. Sex tune-ups may be all you need. If your life includes little kids or a big career, several jobs, or a demanding schedule, this may be the way to take the time that you want with your partner.

Planning another weekend retreat shouldn't be seen as a criticism of your sex life together. Rather, it's another opportunity to connect by getting out of the cycle of every-day life. *Schedule another weekend now, and keep schedul-ing them for periodic emotional pick-me-ups.*

Have some fun thinking about what you would like to do on your next getaway. You probably didn't have time to explore all the options offered, so you'll want to review the earlier chapters to see what you missed that you'd both like to try.

On future sexy getaways, you might want to try any of these additional exercises. We've included some ideas that are a bit exotic, because now that you've made it through the first weekend you could be ready for a little more ad-vanced love play.

Touching and Other Good Vibrations

Start gently on one area of the genitals. Pay special at-tention to the head and under the head of his penis, then lightly touch his scrotal and anal area, which can be highly erotic. While she is stimulating him, he is touching her outer lips and clitoris. He may put his finger inside her vagina, or if she likes anal stimulation, he can gently insert a lubricated finger. To make this exercise more "ad-vanced," both partners can take turns or stimulate each other with two small to medium-size vibrators. Good Vi-brations sells a small vibrator they call the Pocket Rocket, which is 4" long and ⅞" in diameter; the company also sells the Apollo, which is 6" long and 1¼" in diameter.

Vibrators can vary greatly in length and diameter. Check out what is comfortable. The vibrator can be used gently on the penis and in or around the anal area. For women, use one on the outside, near the clitoris, and the other inside the vagina or anus. *Partners sharing sex toys should thoroughly wash them, and always wash toys after using them near the anus.* Used gently and with a lot of feedback from your partner about what feels good, these sex aids can definitely drive both men and women wild.

Taking It Off

Start one of your lovemaking sessions as a striptease artist. Each partner can do this on a separate night as a "show" for the other; having a couple of drinks helps loosen inhibitions. This is one of those rare times when a red lightbulb creates just the right effect. Dress in sexy under-things. Women can buy some incredible stuff through mail-order catalogues, such as see-through body suits and bras that make a woman look as if she is offering up her breasts for nibbling just by taking her shirt off. Put on whatever music you like—hard rock or rhythm and blues is nice background for this game. The partner who is doing the striptease will get excited by acting out this fantasy role.

This scenario does not require having a perfect body. You know what your bodies look like by now. The way you move your body and the sheer fact that you are taking this time to arouse each other are the real turn-ons. Take it slow. Remember, pros go through several layers of clothes and always have a few surprises for the audience. Men, you can wear bikini underwear under your shorts, or strip down to your shorts and stroke yourself so that your partner sees your erection while you're dancing. If dancing is embarrassing for either of you, just walk around seductively to the music. You'll be amazed at how erotic this can be.

Women have the advantage in this exercise. They can

wear more revealing clothes that help set the mood, and they have more experience in drawing attention to their bodies. On the other hand, women are often more embarrassed and distracted by what they consider their physical imperfections. Play the role of someone who knows she is devastatingly sexy and you will overcome your inhibitions.

Slowly move your hands over every part of your body that you uncover—touch each nipple, cup your hands over your breasts and stroke them, and dip your finger inside your vagina. Invent moves as you go along. Turn your back to him and grab your own buttocks. Act as though you are ready for sex and you will have a rapt audience.

So Many Positions

It's time for a few more acrobatic positions. Try 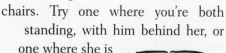 different positions sitting on  chairs. Try one where you're both standing, with him behind her, or one where she is lying on the bed and he is standing and leaning over her. Have him lie on his back and her mount him while on her knees, facing away 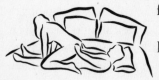 from him. Or partners can both be on their knees on the floor, her knees on top of his as she balances herself with her feet.

Invent new ways to enter and be en-
tered; every angle is a new sensation. We've added a few more
illustrations to spark your
imagination.

"69"
"69" is a challenging position for oral sex. This position
aligns you facing each other's genital area, with the goal of
sucking and licking each other at the same time. There are
two variations: In the first, one partner lies on his or her
back and the other person is on top; in the second, they lie
side by side. If one partner reaches orgasm only on his or
her back, obviously the first position is better, and that
person should be the "bottom" of the couple.

The advantage is simultaneous arousal; the disadvan-
tage is losing your concentration on the other person as
your own excitement becomes overwhelming. You may
want to be pleasure-oriented rather than orgasm-driven in
this position. Reaching orgasm can be difficult, but it is
wonderful when it happens. You can move back to intercourse, or some other activity, when you feel ready to have
an orgasm.

Don't Do This One If You're Going to Run for Public Office
One of the sexiest things you can do is make love in an
unusual place outside the home—on a beach or in an
unlit pool in the summer or in hot springs in the middle of

winter. Though it is probably against airline regulations, plenty of people report that their hottest sex is in the rest room of an airplane. Go camping and put up a tent; rain or shine, there's something really special in making love outside. The awareness that you might be seen is one factor that makes sex in public places really hot, but be sure that you don't put yourself in any danger or risk of being arrested for lewd and lascivious behavior.

Light Bondage and Discipline

We decided to experiment with B&D on this getaway. Using thigh-high nylons as impromptu restraints was totally sexy.

It's not easy (or necessary) to explain why restraints are so sexy for some people, or why imposing your will or submitting to your partner's is such a turn-on. Being "ravished"—well, by the ravisher of your choice—can be thrilling. When playing this game, be sure to take turns. A lot of men like being tied up and ravished, too. You can flip a coin to decide which roles to play—the ravisher or the ravished. Before you start, agree on how long this activity will last. You both need to understand and agree that if either partner gets uncomfortable and says "Stop!" the game ends.

The following scenario is a good beginning: Pretend that the ravisher has been granted three wishes that cannot be refused. Let's say that you've chosen the role of ravisher. Your first wish is that you get to tie up your partner. You can do this with silk scarves, or you can use leather handcuffs.

If you want to make sure no one gets bruised, use soft, fleece-lined Velcro cuffs. Remember, this is just play; no one should get hurt. The person who is being tied up and is submitting to the other's wishes really controls the action. This game has got to be consensual; otherwise, it's abusive.

What are your other two wishes? Do you want to sexually "torture" your victim by turning him on and denying any orgasm until he begs for it? Do you want to leave one hand free, then "order" your partner to masturbate to climax? Or, if she's the slave, you may want her to lie facedown and enter her from behind.

Maybe while your partner is positioned rump up and very turned on, you can start lightly spanking, if you know for sure she or he would think it's fun. Try just one light smack, and see what the response is. If your partner gives clear feedback that this is exciting, you can slap again. Gradually increase intensity with the flat of your hand on the lower buttocks. The partner being spanked tells the other when it's hard enough and when to stop. If this is new territory for you, take it slowly and be sure your partner consents enthusiastically—otherwise, stop.

In such "dominance" play you want to get in touch with pleasing by controlling. In fact, you're allowing your partner to be wildly absorbed in his or her own pleasure. When you're the one being tied up, you're being ordered to do sexual things. You bear no responsibility. Being controlled can be a source of freedom and excitement.

Of course, this kind of experimentation requires a lot of trust. Don't try these games if you are not absolutely sure that bondage and discipline can be safe and non-threatening for both of you.

Gender-Bending

Have you ever wanted to pretend you are a member of the opposite sex? This idea might disgust you—or intrigue you. If the latter is true, go for it. If you are a man, dress up in a nightie or teddy and be seduced by your female partner, who acts out her version of how a guy would do it. To keep in character, the gender-bending man has to be conventionally "on the bottom," the woman, "on top."

If you are a woman, get into the idea of controlling the action and being forceful and directive. If he wants, you can "enter" him with a finger or small vibrator. For the truly daring, a woman can use a strap-on dildo (available at sex boutiques and through mail-order catalogs). Caution: Both partners have to consider themselves real boundary breakers!

Old House, New Places

She sat on the counter in the bathroom and we made love, watching our reflections in the mirror.

Look around your home. Are there places where you've never made love? The kitchen floor? Your desk? In front of the fireplace? On top of the dryer? Your kid's swing set? Get playful. Use your imagination and have some outrageous fun.

SPECIAL VACATIONS

Don't forget that a new location can make repeating the same getaway feel totally different. If you had a fabulous experience at home, try to imagine it taking place in Puerto Vallarta, the Bahamas, or Las Vegas—or the world's sleaziest motor inn, or a cabin in the woods. All these locations have something to offer—each one will bring out a different aspect of the experience.

> *The program did a wonderful thing for us: It allowed us to reclaim our home as a safe haven. Life is so busy that we had become very task-oriented and forgotten how to rest. It's okay to waste time at home. Two Sundays after our "sex holiday" we watched a golf tournament, made love in the afternoon, then took a nap together. Our home is a wonderful place again.*

> *This book is like battery cables. Everyone should have it handy to jump-start their love life!*

An Invitation to Our Readers

We'd love to know what you liked the best about your first getaway and what you look forward to in your future sex getaways. Contact us by mail in care of:

Dr. Pepper Schwartz
The Great Sex Weekend
P.O. Box 2005
Snoqualmie, WA 98096
or send us E-mail: greatsex@greatsexweekend.com
For information and updates, visit our web site:
www.greatsexweekend.com

A 24-Hour Plan

The 24-Hour Plan was really perfect for us. I think most people with two jobs and two kids don't really get much more time than this.

WE RECOGNIZE THAT SOME COUPLES NEED AN abbreviated plan if they are to participate at all. For them, we have included two different one-day plans. We've highlighted some of the exercises and activities from the weekend getaway that we think will be most beneficial to couples who want to jump-start their sex lives in a very short time.

PLAN ONE: SATURDAY MORNING UNTIL SUNDAY MORNING

The first short program is intended for those who are staying at home and devoting a full Saturday to each other. Here we provide only the rudimentary outline of the plan and include reference to pages in previous chapters that offer more detail.

BREAKFAST IN BED. This luxury is the earliest and easiest way to signal that today is special. Take turns pampering each other; one partner prepares breakfast in bed on Saturday, the other on Sunday. (See pp. 78–79, for specific suggestions.)

BATHING TOGETHER. Take a sensual shower or bath together. (See pp. 79–80, for playful bathing ideas.)

EXCHANGING FULL-BODY MASSAGES. While you're in the mood to spoil your partner and be spoiled yourself, we recommend that you consult pp. 104–106 to learn about how to relax and enjoy the intimacy of swapping massages. We also suggest trying the pleasuring exercises (described on pp. 63–64), which will show you how to incorporate giving and getting feedback into your massage experience. Like pleasuring, massage helps you rediscover the full range of erotic stimulation, but it is also an occasion to communicate with each other how you are feeling and how you want to be touched.

SADIE HAWKINS DAY. By reversing many of the traditional male and female roles, women can more readily become the sexual initiator. Among other suggestions, we encourage women to select new, exciting positions for intercourse. Four positions are described on pp. 85–91, along with some tips for making the Sadie Hawkins concept work for you.

AFTERNOON BREAK. We don't expect or recommend that you stay in bed all day. Instead of the all-afternoon break described in chapter 4, a two-hour break fits this plan better. Some of the suggested activities listed on pp. 91–92 are suitable, or you can simply take a leisurely walk or drive. Weather permitting, pack a picnic lunch and head to a relaxing outdoor setting. A long lunch at a restaurant with a beautiful view is a good second choice.

TOUCHING OR ORAL SEX TO CLIMAX. The "his and her" exercises described on pp. 65–74 remind you that all sex doesn't have to be centered around intercourse. You can bring each other to an exciting orgasm with your hands and mouth.

ROLE-PLAYING AT DINNER. If you think it would be enjoyable, step out of your own lives and into a sexy, romantic "play" at dinner where you each take the lead roles. See pp. 98–101 and 108–109 for ideas and cautionary notes.

ALTERNATE DINNER EXERCISE—INTIMATE TALK. On pp. 59–60 and 119–122, you'll find suggestions for romantic and sexy topics that will tease and tantalize. You may never make it to dessert.

SEX ON A SATURDAY NIGHT. For those of you who engaged in fantasy role-playing at dinner, stay in character. Sex automatically takes on a fresh and different flavor when you're pretending to be someone. Your post-dinner lovemaking can be very exciting.

If you didn't indulge in a fantasy scenario, you may prefer to try out a new sex toy (see pp. 118–119), swap fantasies or sex checks (see pp. 45, 95–97), paint each other's body (see pp. 109–111), or watch an adult video (see pp. 107–108). Any of these props should also lead you to out-of-the ordinary sexual fun.

RELAX WITH A ROMANTIC MOVIE. It's nice to relax and snuggle after sex. Pick a light romantic comedy or drama that you enjoyed together in the past but haven't seen in years. For those who'd like to try something a little sexier, consult the list of R-rated films touted by *Playboy* for their "searing movie scenes" (see pp. 102–103).

SUNDAY MORNING. This is the last breakfast in bed, or brunch on the patio, before reentry to everyday life. Write each other a brief letter about the highlights of your mini-getaway. Jot down your feelings about your relationship and your partner (see pp. 123–125). Exchange and talk about your letters. If you want to go further, explore some of the issues touched upon on pp. 127–130—this process can help you bring extra excitement into your everyday erotic life. You might discuss what you'd like to do on your next getaway.

Plan Two: Saturday Afternoon to Sunday Afternoon

The second short program is intended for those who can get away from home. It conforms to most late-afternoon check-in and noon checkout times. Here we offer a rudimentary outline of the plan and reference to pages in previous chapters that offer more detail.

An Intimate Lunch. You can request early check-in privileges, but we're assuming you'll have to wait until after lunch to get into most hotels. When you reach your destination, have lunch in the prettiest restaurant on the premises or in the nearby vicinity. Consult the list of suggested romantic or sexy conversation topics described on pp. 59–60 and 119–122 that will put you in the mood for the twenty-four hours ahead.

Afternoon Nooky. Following your intimate lunch, you probably can't wait to get to your room. We recommend that you carefully read about the postdinner activities described on pp. 60–65. For the afternoon adaptation, start by undressing each other (this can be slow and teasing or fast and desperate) and doing the kissing exercise. Skip the pleasuring exercise and move directly to the eye-contact exercise, which involves touching, looking, and talking. From there, as you'll see, you are encouraged to pleasure each other with some combination of touching, oral and even anal stimulation, as well as intercourse to orgasm, as you like it.

BATHING TOGETHER. After sex, take a sensual shower or bath together. See pp. 79–80 for suggestions. If it's already getting dark, you might consider taking a candlelit bath. See pp. 103 for ideas about how to enhance your bath. If the hotel has a Jacuzzi, this might be a nice time to enjoy that relaxing activity together.

SHORT WALK AND TALK. This is an easy activity to do just about anywhere you go, but if you feel the need for more exercise, see what the hotel or area offers. You don't need to indulge in a full workout. The important thing is to be together.

COCKTAILS, DINNER, AND FANTASY. If you think it would be enjoyable, we recommend stepping out of your own lives and into a sexy, romantic "play" for predinner cocktails. This role-playing should carry you through dinner. Read pp. 98–101 for ideas and cautionary notes. A "pickup" or "first meeting" scene is the easiest to enact in a public place.

RELAX WITH AN IN-ROOM MOVIE. Select a sexy drama or a romantic comedy. Relax and snuggle or have more sex. This should be a low-key prelude to a long, deep sleep together.

Breakfast in Bed. Call for room service and indulge yourselves in this out-of-the-ordinary luxury.

Sadie Hawkins Day. A little role reversal can bring added excitement to any relationship, so we encourage the woman to take on the role of sexual initiator (see pp. 81–85). We suggest that she select positions for intercourse that she has never explored before. Four positions are described on pp. 85–91.

Last Stroll or Lunch. Before you return to everyday life, write each other a brief letter about the highlights of your mini-getaway. Include feelings about your relationship and your partner (see pp. 123–125). Exchange and talk about your letters. If you want to go further, you can have a conversation based on the questions posed on pp. 127–130 that can help you improve your everyday erotic life. You might include what you'd like to do on your next getaway.

> *We had too much anxiety about getting away for two days. One day was perfect. No guilt. No regrets. We think we should do the one-day getaway at least once a month.*

APPENDIX 2

Getaway Places

THIS IS NOT AN EXHAUSTIVE LIST OF CITIES OR hotels, just some ideas of places we like and think you might like too. Some hotels were suggested by road-test couples; others are ones that we personally have known and loved. Some hotels and inns have offered discounts, little gifts, or extra services to couples doing our program; we suggest that you mention our book in those places.

It's hard to rate hotels according to price—everyone has a different notion of what is considered expensive. Also, certain cities operate on a different scale. For example, what is reasonable in New York City is considered expensive almost everywhere else. So here is our general approach: If a room is under $100, or close to it, we call it inexpensive. If it is between $100 and $200, we call it moderate. If it is over $200, we say it is expensive. (The one exception to this formula is New York City, where a moderately priced room can cost approximately $225.)

National Hotel Chains: In addition to the city-by-city list that follows, the major hotel chains offer "romance packages" subject to availability (there is some variation according to individual hotel). For example, Marriott offers "Weekends for Two," with free breakfast in bed, 25 percent off dinner, and late Sunday checkout. Call 800-USA-WKND. Hilton's "Romance Package" typically includes breakfast, a bottle of champagne or sparkling cider, bubble bath, and chocolate-covered strawberries. Call 800-HILTONS. Hyatt's "Romance Packages" are less generous, but call 800-233-1234 and inquire about details.

*U*NITED *S*TATES

Atlanta

Ritz Carlton—Buckhead   3434 Peachtree Road Northeast (ZIP 30326)   404-237-2700; fax: 404-239-0078 This hotel doesn't look like the classic Ritz Carlton from the outside, but inside it is all paneling and flowers and oil paintings. The good news is that it's a better price than most and includes all their usual amenities, like terrific service and a good health club. There is a very fancy, romantic restaurant and a great open bar for people-watching. The rooms are romantic, and when you take your break, there are some great shopping plazas right across the street. Moderate to expensive.

Grand Hyatt   3300 Peachtree Road (ZIP 30305) 404-365-8100; fax: 404-233-5686.   If you like the elegance of simple but luxurious Japanese ambience, this is the place for you. There are beautiful Japanese gardens to stroll through and rooms that are tasteful and spacious. We like the attention to details: marble bathrooms with thick terry robes, 24-hour room service, and fine service. Moderate to expensive.

Chateau Elan   100 Rue Charlegmagne, Braselton (ZIP 30517)   800-233-WINE or 770-932-0900   This is a large resort with a spa, golf course, tennis courts, and riding facilities. The European ambience includes a very serious approach to food. We recommend it because many of the suites have been built to house honeymooners. But the rooms vary widely, so be specific about what you are looking for. Moderate.

Boston

Ritz-Carlton   15 Arlington Street (ZIP 02117) 617-536-5700   This is one of the nicest hotels in the whole chain. Want to be pampered? Want to feel special? Look no further. The French public rooms are exquisite, and your room is likely to be lovely, too. There is limousine service upon request—in fact, you ask, and they deliver. Not surprisingly, expensive.

Boston Harbor Hotel   70 Rowes Wharf (ZIP 02110)   617-439-7000; fax: 617-330-9450   What a wonderful place to get away to. This hotel has large bedrooms with large baths, and the public rooms feel celebratory. For a break, there is a spa and indoor pool, and at night their lounge offers good jazz. Moderate to expensive.

The Newbury Guest House   261 Newbury Street (ZIP 02116)   617-437-7666   This is Victorian Boston, a four-story town house built in 1882. Some people think it's Boston's best lodging—at any price. There is a wonderfully cozy atmosphere and a great location. Inexpensive to moderate.

Regal Bostonian Hotel at Faneuil Hall Marketplace,   24 North Street (ZIP 02109)   617-523-3600; fax: 617-523-2454   This place feels like a small urban inn, even though it has 152 rooms. There are balconies and French doors and French furniture, all of which add up to a very romantic atmosphere. Some of the rooms have fireplaces; all have VCRs, oversize bathtubs, and terry robes. Moderate to expensive.

. . . . *Near Boston*

CAMBRIDGE
The Charles Hotel   One Bennett Street (ZIP 02138) 617-864-1200; fax: 617-864-5715   This is a charming medium-size hotel with inviting rooms that tell you you are in New England. We especially like the quilted down

comforters. There is 24-hour room service and a health club and spa. Moderate to expensive.

MARTHA'S VINEYARD

Captain R. Flander's House North Road, P.O. Box 384, Chilmark (ZIP 02535) 508-645-3123 This is a lovely bed-and-breakfast in a historic house on lovely acreage overlooking Bliss Pond. Reeks Martha Stewart—in fact, she featured it in one of her books. It is small. The best place for lovers is the separate cottage with fireplace. Very romantic. Moderate.

Outermost Inn 171 Lighthouse Road, Aquinnah (ZIP 02535) 508-645-3511 If your idea of romance is a classic Vineyard shingled house on a bluff overlooking the sea, search no more. There is a first-rate restaurant, lovely rooms (including one suite), and simple romantic decoration. Expensive.

Thorncroft Inn 460 Main Street, Vineyard Haven (ZIP 02568) 508-693-3333 More laid-back than some of the others. You can stay in the main inn or in a remodeled carriage house. Less family oriented, so better for lovers—especially the private hot tubs, which can be reserved. Moderate.

Central California Coast

Sycamore Mineral Springs Resort 1215 Avila Beach Drive, San Luis Obispo (ZIP 93405) 800-234-5831 or

805-595-7302; fax: 805-781-2598   This is a natural hot springs resort located on a hillside, only three minutes from the beach. Each room features a full-size spa and private balcony, suites have fireplaces, oversize showers, and four-poster beds. Other spa amenities offered. Romantic restaurant on premises. Mention our book. Moderate to expensive.

Ripplewood Inn   Hwy 1, Big Sur (ZIP 93920) 831-667-2242   Individual heated redwood cabins, most with kitchens and fireplaces. Some have two bedrooms and private decks. Inexpensive.

The Madonna Inn   100 Madonna Road, San Luis Obispo (ZIP 93405)   800-543-9666 or 805-543-3000; fax: 805-543-1800   109 different rooms, ranging from one with seven-foot bathtub, another has a cave room theme with a waterfall shower, then there's a hearts-and-flowers for the truly sentimental. This is only for couples with a sense of humor. Be prepared for hordes of tourists; this place is kitschy fun. Moderate.

Charleston

27 State Street Bed-and-Breakfast   (ZIP 29401) 843-722-4243   Built in 1800 in the French Quarter, this old private residence now has suites with private entrances, some with fireplaces and kitchens. Flowers and fruit in the room. Beach close by. Inexpensive to moderate.

Middleton Inn   Ashley River Road (ZIP 29414) 800-543-4774 or 843-556-0500   On a fabulous old plantation. Play Rhett and Scarlett. Great grounds for holding hands and romance. Lovely, classic furnishings. Privacy. Moderate to expensive.

John Rutledge House   116 Broad Street (ZIP 29401)   843-723-7999   Antebellum mansion on the Historic Register. An old ballroom with wrought-iron staircases is locale for tea and sherry in the afternoon. Poster beds and lavish baths, two with Jacuzzis. Marble fireplaces in some rooms. Inexpensive to moderate.

Chicago

The Drake   140 East Walton Place (ZIP 60611) 800-553-7253; fax: 312-787-2549   This is a Chicago institution, and it looks a little bit like a place where ladies lunch. But you are right across from a wonderful beach and can turn the corner to some of the best walking/shopping streets in the world. If you get a room with a water view, it can be spectacular. As with other older, venerable hotels you have to request a good room that's big enough. A lot of class, and service. Moderate to expensive.

Sutton Place Hotel   21 East Bellevue Place (ZIP 60611)   312-266-2100; fax: 312-266-2103   This is right in the center of the Gold Coast near Lake Michigan, and it is a handsome place. There is art deco decoration and big rooms with VCRs, CD players, and great sound systems.

The bathrooms are a special plus; they are large, and each one has a soaking tub with a separate shower. Twenty-four-hour room service, of course. Moderate to expensive.

The Four Seasons Hotel   120 East Delaware Place (ZIP 60611)   312-280-8800; fax: 312-280-1748   If you want a splurge getaway, do it here. The lobby is on the seventh floor, and when you walk in you feel as if you are in an especially luxurious place. The rooms with a view of the skyline or Lake Michigan are terrific. Expensive.

The Talbot   20 East Delaware Place (ZIP 60611) 312-944-4970 or 800-621-8506   This is a real find on the Gold Coast. Based on the personal approach of a European hotel, this hotel specializes in romance and offers Suite Dreams Weekends, which feature champagne, flowers, and a one-bedroom suite and Sunday brunch. Paneled public rooms with fireplaces and room service when you want it. Moderate.

. . . . *Near Chicago*

UNION PIER
Pine Garth Inn   15790 Union Pier (ZIP 49129) 616-469-1642   There was a time when Union Pier was the place for families from Detroit or Chicago to go. Then it fell on hard times, but once again there is new and post-yuppie interest in creating wonderful spots to go. This one is adult oriented, peaceful, and perfect for a romantic getaway. Fresh flowers and complimentary candy—

champagne for special occasions. It is on the lake, with a private beach to hold hands on. Mention our book for a weekend discount. Inexpensive to moderate.

UTICA
Starved Rock Lodge   Route 71 & 178 Starved Rock State Park (ZIP 61373) 815-667-4211   This is a rustic lodge in beautiful scenery about one and a half hours from Chicago. The pine-paneled lodge has some rooms with fireplaces, an indoor pool, and wonderful walks along the Illinois River. Inexpensive to moderate.

MEQUON
Sybaris   10240 Cedarburg Road (ZIP 53092) 414-242-8000 On a beautifully landscaped 10-acre site along the Milwaukee River, this country inn hideaway is part of the Sybaris chain that specializes in romantic getaways for married couples. Award-winning restaurant. Sybaris suites feature in-room swimming pools and whirlpool spas with extras like lots of mirrors. There are three other locations in the Chicago area. Inexpensive to expensive.

Dallas

Adolphus Hotel   1321 Commerce Street (ZIP 75202) 800-221-9083 or 214-742-8200; fax: 214-651-3561   This hotel has an elegant English atmosphere. The bedrooms have four-posters and are tastefully decorated. For atmosphere, try the afternoon tea. Moderate to expensive.

The Mansion on Turtle Creek   2821 Turtle Creek Boulevard (ZIP 75219)   214-559-2100; fax: 214-528-4187   This is the place to eat and sleep in Dallas. All the amenities: marble baths, terry robes, and more service than you will know what to do with. There is an outdoor swimming pool and a health club. Expensive.

The Dallas Medallion   4099 Valley View Lane (ZIP 75244)   972-385-9000; fax: 972-788-1174   This hotel has been redecorated and now is a lovely place to curl up in. The bedrooms are very large and have big, comfy chairs. Twenty-four-hour room service and reasonable prices. Moderate.

Denver

Loews Giorgio Hotel   4150 East Mississippi Avenue (ZIP 80246)   800-345-9172 or 303-782-9300; fax: 303-758-6542   This hotel has an Italian theme; the public rooms make you feel as if you were in a villa. The suites shine here, and the regular rooms are not as special. A little bit away from downtown in the Cherry Creek district—which helps you feel a bit more away from it all. Moderate.

The Oxford Hotel   1600 Seventeenth Street (ZIP 80202)   800-228-5838 or 303-628-5400; fax: 303-628-5413   This historic hotel features English and French antiques, marble floors, and stained glass. Located just off the Sixteenth Street Mall and Tabor Center and within walking distance of Coors Field and art galleries. Ask about their romance packages. Moderate to expensive.

Holtze Executive Suites 818 Seventeenth Street
(ZIP 80202)   800-422-2092 or 303-607-9000; fax: 303-
607-0101   These suites offer a lot of privacy and include
a comfortable living room with fireplaces and fully
equipped kitchen. Complimentary breakfast and health
club on-site. Walking distance of Sixteenth Street Mall.
Moderate.

. . . . *Near Denver*

BOULDER
Hotel Boulderado 2115 13th Street (ZIP 80302)
800-433-4344 or 303-442-4344; fax: 303-442-4378
Victorian elegance. 160 guest rooms and suites. Features
magnificent views of Boulder and the Rocky Mountains.
One block from award-winning pedestrian mall. Beautiful
and bustling. Moderate.

ASPEN
Want to splurge? Choose the Little Nell (675 East
Durant [ZIP 81611]   970-920-4600), which has good
rates off season. Pretty rooms—both right near the slopes
(the Little Nell is practically on them) and in the middle
of a wonderful walking town. Out of our usual driving
range—but, of course, worth it.

VAIL
Half the distance from Denver and a great village en-
vironment at Vail and at Beaver Creek. Both have nice ex-
amples of good chain hotels—the Sheraton, Westin, the
Hyatt, etc.—and the scenery is scrumptious.

The Lodge and Spa at Cordillera   P.O. Box 1110 Edwards, Vail Valley (ZIP 81632)   970-926-2200; fax: 970-926-2486   A really nice chateau-style lodge and spa. About twenty minutes from Vail in a beautiful setting with lots of privacy. All the rooms have lovely views of the mountains from their own balconies or terraces. Take your breaks at the health club, relaxing in the sauna or steam room or in an indoor heated lap pool. Choose from indoor and outdoor hot tubs. Moderate to expensive.

Houston

La Columb d'Or   3410 Montrose Boulevard (ZIP 77006)   713-524-7999   If you like the feeling of being pampered in your own mansion, come here. Only six rooms, each individually decorated with French themes. The nice part of this place is that they will cater to you, but they will also let you alone—perfect for our purposes. Elegant and expensive—but not over the top.

South Shore Harbor Resort and Conference Center 2500 South Shore Boulevard, Leigh City (ZIP 77573) 800-442-5005 or 281-334-1000; fax: 281-334-1157   A nice getaway drive from Houston, just about halfway to Galveston. Right on the harbor, and most rooms have water views. The rooms are simple but nice. There is a fitness center, which has a lap pool and also a big Hawaii-type pool with a waterfall and a bar you can swim up to. There is also a boat center, and you can rent a sailboat or even go fishing. Quite moderate to expensive.

Angel Arbor Bed-and-Breakfast 921 Heights Boulevard (ZIP 77008-6911) 713-868-4654 This Victorian is on the National Historic Register, and it's a nice change of pace. There is a solarium and a gazebo and those other Victoria's Secret romantic touches. Make sure you get one of the rooms with a private bath! Inexpensive.

Los Angeles

The Argyle 8358 Sunset Boulevard, West Hollywood (ZIP 90069) 323-654-7100; fax: 323-654-9287 Wonderful skyline views from the pool and one-bedroom suites and great rooms, all with marble bathrooms and many with Jacuzzis. If you like art deco splendor and a trendy venue, this is the place to go. Moderate to expensive.

Chateau Marmont 8221 West Sunset Boulevard, Hollywood (ZIP 90046) 323-656-1010 Grab yourself a bit of history. There are 63 suites, but if you can, reserve one of those very private bungalows. There is a pool, fitness center, and lots of people-watching, since this is a place where Hollywood film people congregate. If you like "old Hollywood," this place will turn you on. Moderate to expensive.

The Inn at Playa del Rey 435 Culver Boulevard, Playa del Rey (ZIP 90293) 310-574-1920; fax: 310-574-9920 Right at the edge of a bird sanctuary, and definitely designed for lovers. Lavish breakfast, bikes to use on the 30-mile bike path that goes along the ocean, and an outdoor Jacuzzi. Ask for a queen- or king-size bed and a room with a whirlpool bath and fireplace. Some have decks overlooking the marina, and there are "romance suites" that feature king-size canopy beds. Mention the book here. Inexpensive to expensive (includes breakfast).

. . . . *Near Los Angeles*

CATALINA

Hotel Vista del Mar   417 Crescent Avenue, Avalon (ZIP 90704)   310-510-1452   This is a small, wonderful hotel with 13 rooms and two suites. Some of the rooms have hot tubs and fireplaces. We think the island itself is romantic, and just going there can get your blood racing. This hotel places you on the beach with a view of pretty Avalon Bay. Inexpensive to expensive.

Inn at Mount Ada   398 Wrigley Road, Avalon (ZIP 90704)   310-510-2030   If you are looking for something really special, stay in the former home of the Wrigley family. There are only a few rooms, so you have to book way ahead, but you are really living the life of a millionaire here. Expensive.

LAGUNA BEACH.

Surf and Sand Hotel   1555 South Coast Highway (ZIP 92651) 800-664-7873; fax: 949-494-2897   Perched over the sea, this romantic spot makes you feel like you are on the Mediterranean. Flowers everywhere, garden walkways, and private patios. Moderate.

MALIBU

Malibu Beach Inn   22878 Pacific Coast Highway (ZIP 90265)   310-456-6445; fax: 310-456-1499   This is the perfect place for a romantic interlude. It is right on the water, and all the bedrooms have a full or partial view. There are tile baths and fireplaces, and a cute lobby with tea or coffee. Has just the right feel for a tryst. Moderate to expensive.

SANTA MONICA

Shangri-la Hotel   1301 Ocean Avenue (ZIP 90401)   310-394-2791; fax: 310-451-3351   Across the street from the Pacific Ocean, this Steamship Deco small hotel offers a romantic garden patio and two penthouse suites, each with its own balcony. In-room refrigerators. Ten percent discount to our readers who show the book, with box of chocolates upon arrival. Moderate.

Shutters on the Beach   1 Pico Boulevard (ZIP 90405)   800-334-9000 or 310-458-0030; fax: 310-458-4589   The regular rooms are small, but the suites are nice and there are also a pool, hot tub, and fitness center. The views are wonderful. We think this is a fun escape, right next to the boardwalk. Expensive.

PALM SPRINGS AND OTHER
DESERT DESTINATIONS

Two Bunch Palms Trail   67-425 Two Bunch Palms Trail, Desert Hot Springs (ZIP 92240)   760-329-8791 The two of you can go here and pretend to be movie stars.

There are hot tubs and rock and waterfall pools, and several other ways to pamper your body. We like it for the sexy places to relax or walk, and the privacy. Moderate to expensive.

La Mancha Private Villas and Spa, Palm Springs 444 N. Avenuenida Caballeros (ZIP 92262) 1-888-LAMANCHA   This place offers both rooms and suites, but get the latter. There are two mineral pools, plus a regular pool and hot tub. Inexpensive to moderate.

Marriott Desert Springs Resort and Spa 74855 Country Club Drive, Palm Desert (ZIP 92260) 800-331-3112   This is a huge place—with three pools, several fine restaurants, champion golf courses, tennis, and European spa. The rooms are very nice, and many of them open into suites with full kitchens. There is a dramatic lake and canals that some people love and others find too weird in the desert. Fabulous landscaping. Moderate to expensive.

RIVERSIDE
Mission Inn 3649 Mission Inn Avenue (ZIP 92501) 800-843-7755   This is a large place, but they cater to romantic weekends and have some real bargains, such as combining a night in a suite with dinner, two massages, champagne, etc. There are beautiful grounds to walk, too. Moderate to expensive.

SANTA BARBARA
El Encanto Hotel and Garden Villas 1900 Lasuen Road (ZIP 93103) 805-687-5000   There are villas and

cottages, a pool, tennis courts, and a charming town to visit. This place is very private and romantic. Moderate to moderately expensive.

Montecito Inn 1295 Coast Village Road (ZIP 93108) 800-843-2017 or 805-969-7854 Very close to Santa Barbara but known in its own right—and for good reason. This lovely place has charming suites and rooms. Many of the suites come with hot tubs, and the whole atmosphere is private and civilized. Moderate to expensive.

VENTURA AND OXNARD
Mandalay Beach Resort 2101 Mandalay Beach Road, Oxnard (ZIP 93035) 805-985-2500 or 800-EMBASSY Only one hour to paradise. 250 suites right on the beach. Tennis, swimming, spas, complimentary full breakfast and cocktails included. Moderate to expensive.

Inn on the Beach 1175 South Seaward Avenue, Ventura (ZIP 93001) 805-652-2000 Enjoy sunsets from your balcony. This is the only hotel in Ventura that is right on the sand. Not fancy, but a good value and great hideaway. All rooms with fireplaces. Refrigerators available upon request. Inexpensive to moderate.

Miami Beach

The Kent 1131 Collins (ZIP 33139) 800-688-7678 or 305-531-6771 All the amenities for a song. Collins Avenue has been reclaimed and there is now a stylish scene—and the Kent's sophisticated decor is part of this renaissance. Inexpensive.

The Tides 1220 Ocean Drive (ZIP 33139)   800-688-7678   This is a wonderful art deco restoration. There are now 45 suites with 1930s style and flair. A nice touch are blackout curtains for sleeping in and a pool that accommodates topless bathing. It is on the beach, with views from every room. Moderate to very expensive.

The Albion—South Beach 1650 James Avenue (ZIP 33160) 305-913-1000   This beach hotel has a very nautical theme. There are even six three-walled suites that are open to the ocean. It's very high tech, with touches like porthole windows that let you look into the pool. The rooms are simple but airy. Moderate.

. . . . *Near Miami Beach*

BOCA RATON
The Boca Raton Resort and Club   501 E. Camino Real (ZIP 33431-0825)   800-327-0100 or 561-395-3000; fax: 561-447-3183   This is really a group of hotels, the "old money" pink historic Cloister, the sleek Tower, and the casual Beach Club—which is right on the water. There is a shuttle that takes you from one to the other—so if you stay at one you don't have to miss the others entirely! We recommend staying at the older hotel and visiting the beach by shuttle service—after all, you won't be

out of doors that much. Moderate with a few expensive options.

FORT LAUDERDALE
The Riverside Hotel 620 East Las Olas Boulevard 800-325-3280; fax: 305-462-2148 This is the perfect get-away find, overlooking the river and boats. The place is "old Florida," but this is not a formal, elegant getaway—rather, it is full of warm ambience for a reasonable price. Mostly suites, inviting and casual. Inexpensive to moderate.

PALM BEACH
The Breakers One South County Road (ZIP 33480) 561-655-6611; fax: 561-659-8403 This is the real thing. Italian Renaissance splendor modeled on the Villa Medici in Rome, this time on the ocean in an idyllic scene for romance. The rooms, we are assured, are sound-proof. VCRs and refrigerators can be rented. Special romance packages. Expensive.

Minneapolis
Nicolet Island Inn 95 Merriam Street (ZIP 55401) 612-331-1800 This is a small renovated inn located on a river island near the center of Minneapolis. The rooms are cozy, decorated with antique furniture, and the lobby is welcoming, with a fireplace and cozy restaurant. For a break, consider the nearby park. Inexpensive to moderate.

Doubletree Guest Suites   1101 LaSalle Avenue (ZIP 55403)   612-332-6800; fax: 612-232-8246   We are partial to suite hotels because they give us a little breathing room and also, sometimes, some kitchen facilities. This one had a wet bar and a room refrigerator and the usual amenities. Not fancy, but nice, with a dignified lobby. Inexpensive to moderate.

New England
. . . . In Connecticut

WESTPORT
The Inn at National Hall   2 Post Road West (ZIP 06880)   203-221-1351   This is an historic hotel, very beautiful, very much interested in pampering you. Truly elegant, formal decoration. Bedrooms and suites with canopy beds, little sitting areas, antiques. One hour away from Manhattan. Moderate to expensive.

MYSTIC
The Inn at Mystic   Routes 1 and 27 (ZIP 06355) 800-237-2415 or 860-536-9604   This has all sorts of accommodations; some are deluxe with balconies that view the harbor, others are not so special. You have to do a little investigative work to make sure you get something really romantic, but they are to be had—after all, we have heard that this is where Bogie and Lauren Bacall spent their honeymoon. Moderate to expensive.

NORWALK

Silvermine Tavern 194 Perry Avenue (ZIP 06850) 203-847-4558 Small. Charming, in the middle of antiquing countryside. Several of the rooms have fireplaces. There is a serious waterfall to listen to, and it seems the perfect place to get away to for a lovely weekend. It is popular, however (both the inn and the restaurant), so reserve far in advance. Inexpensive to moderate.

. . . . *In Maine*

Captain Lord Mansion P.O. Box 800, Kennebunkport (ZIP 04046) 207-967-3141; fax: 207-967-3172 These lavishly decorated rooms have canopied beds and fireplaces—one deluxe suite even has a large multijet shower and a Jacuzzi-type bath. The town is bustling in the summer, but it's a wonderful, quiet escape out of season. Inexpensive to expensive.

The Inn at Harbor Head 41 Pier Road, Kennebunkport (ZIP 04046) 207-967-5564 This might be just what you are looking for—elegantly artistic furnishings and rooms with Jacuzzis, terry robes, and fireplaces, and all that right next to the waterfront. Moderate to expensive.

The Inn at Sunrise Point Route 1, Camden (ZIP 04849) 207-236-7716 This romantic location is near Camden. The very nice rooms are on the water—but even nicer, there are some very private cottages. Most of them have Jacuzzi bathtubs and fireplaces. Moderate to expensive.

. . . . *In New Hampshire*

Adair, Bethlehem   80 Guider Lane, Bethlehem (ZIP 03574)   603-444-2600   This is a 200-acre estate originally designed by the famous Olmsted Brothers, who also designed Central Park in New York City. There is great service, lovely rooms, and wonderful walks. Moderate.

Balsams Grand Resort Hotel   Dixville Notch (ZIP 03576)   800-255-0600   You might find this huge place overwhelming, but it has every service you could possibly want. It is nestled into the hills on the water, and the vast acreage asks you to wander it. Expensive.

. . . . *In Vermont*

Jackson House   481 Woodstock Road, Woodstock (ZIP 05091)   802-457-2065   An elegant getaway with great hospitality from the owners. Champagne and appetizers are served in the beautiful garden during good weather. There are both rooms and suites available. Moderate to expensive.

The Inn at Shelburne Farms   1611 Harbor Road, Shelburne (ZIP 05482)   802-985-8498   A striking mansion located on a beautiful farm right at the edge of Lake Champlain. Very romantic. Inexpensive to moderate.

New Orleans

Soniat House   1133 Chartres Street (ZIP 70116) 800-544-8808 or 504-522-0570   This is a truly romantic setting. There is a shaded courtyard lit with candles at night, vines trailing on balconies, and breakfast served in the courtyard. Bedrooms are located in several restored buildings, and the rooms vary from romantic to extraordinary. Moderate to expensive.

Maison De Ville   727 Toulouse Street (ZIP 70130) 800-634-1600 or 504-561-5858   The hotel is very nice, but the real romantic retreats are in the cottages. The cottages are suites, and they have their own garden with a swimming pool in a shared central area. They are so romantic that a lot of other people want to book them, too—so reserve way ahead. There is also a romantic restaurant you probably want to reserve a spot in. Moderate to expensive.

Windsor Court Hotel   300 Grazier Street (ZIP 70130)   800-262-2662 or 504-523-6000   The exterior is modern and not particularly alluring, but you enter through a nice courtyard and the rooms are quite appealing: They all have a sitting area, and most have four-poster beds and traditional furnishings. There is fastidious room service and very fine amenities throughout. Expensive.

New York

The Inn at Irving Place   56 Irving Place (ZIP 10003)   212-533-4600; fax: 212-533-4611   This hotel is in Gramercy Park a little bit off the beaten path. It puts you firmly in nineteenth-century New York. There are twelve guest rooms and suites and many nice touches, like the ability to bring your breakfast back to your room. No young children allowed—which makes this perfect for a couple getaway. Expensive, but not for New York.

The Lowell   28 East Sixty-third Street (ZIP 10021) 212-838-1400 or 800-221-4444   A delightful historic hotel in a lovely, quiet part of New York. Elegant decor, mostly suites, with marble bathrooms, many with fireplaces and small kitchens that are filled with romantic snacks like champagne and cheese. The decorations are old money: chintz, lovely prints, comforters, and antiques. Great service and a romantic tearoom. A special place for lovers. Expensive.

The Plaza at Central Park   Fifty-ninth and Fifth Avenue (ZIP 10019)   800-759-3000 or 212-546-5493 Well, it's the Plaza! There is the wonderful Oak Room for dinner and the Plaza Court for Tea, the horse carriages outside, and the Park for your morning run. It's just about irresistible. The rooms vary a lot, though, so you have to be careful to get a large, cheerful one. Also, because the Plaza is now owned by the Westin, look for deals and special offerings. Expensive.

The Soho Grand   310 West Broadway (ZIP 10013)
800-965-3000 or 212-965-3000   A new hotel. High-tech
with soaring spaces and an attempt to give a new and interesting hotel to the arts capital of New York. They have
succeeded in putting together both a chic and welcoming
place with all the amenities and not too much sticker
shock. Moderate to expensive.

. . . . *Near New York*

THE ADIRONDACKS
Sagamore in the Adirondacks   P.O. Box 146,
Raquette Lake, NY (ZIP 13436)   315-354-5311   This is
one of the classic old "camps" of the rich that is now available to the rest of us—though not inexpensively. Rustic
but romantic—think of yourself canoeing on the lake at
twilight. Cottages are probably the better getaway bet.
Moderate to expensive.

THE HAMPTONS
Hedges Inn   74 James Lane, East Hampton (ZIP
11937)   516-324-7100   A nineteenth-century house
with all those nice New England touches. The rooms are
all done with care—Laura Ashley prints and lovely linens.
For our purposes, get one of the rooms with a fireplace so
you can have a romantic candlelight dinner. Moderate to
expensive.

1770 House   143 Main Street, East Hampton
(ZIP 11937) 516-324-1770   A completely winning place
with a great restaurant. Antiques everywhere, and each

with a great restaurant. Antiques everywhere, and each room has a personality all its own. Some of the rooms are extremely large and luxurious. Moderate to expensive.

Philadelphia

Four Seasons Hotel   1 Logan Square (ZIP 19103) 800-332-3442 or 215-963-1500   This is such a great chain—you can never really go wrong with one of their hotels. They are pricey, though, so look for special rate offerings. They all have an English-style elegance to them, fresh flowers, inventive menus, and usually very nice decoration, amenities, and bathrooms. They pride themselves on service. Expensive.

Park Hyatt Philadelphia   200 South Broad Street (ZIP 19102)   800-233-1234; 215-893-1776; fax: 215-732-8518   Feel truly grand walking in and out of this hotel with classic older-hotel elegance. The rooms vary and can be small, but there are very pretty ones (and pretty good noise protection). There is a great health club. Very Philadelphia. Expensive.

. . . . *Near Philadelphia*

AMISH COUNTRY
Waynebrook Inn   Route 10 and Route 322, Honey Brook (ZIP 19344)   610-273-2444; fax: 610-273-3722 The outside of this hotel is eighteenth century, but the inside is all new. There is an especially romantic dining room with private nooks, perfect for making you feel as if

you are having an affair with each other. Bedrooms are nicely decorated, and some have kitchenettes. Moderate.

BETHLEHEM
Wydnor Hall 3612 Old Philadelphia Pike (ZIP 18015-5320) 610-867-6851 or 800-839-0020; fax: 610-866-2062 Very nice, old-city Georgian house. Elegant public rooms and bedrooms. Wonderful breakfasts. Special attention to details like lovely linens, heated towel racks, and terry-cloth robes. Some suites include a two-person shower that converts to a steam room. Inexpensive to moderate.

BUCKS COUNTY
Maplewood Farm Bed-and-Breakfast 5090 Durham Road, Gardenville (ZIP 18926) 215-766-0477 A beautiful eighteenth-century stone farmhouse on a peaceful five-acre farm. Charming bedrooms that include four-poster beds or a two-story suite with beams and a sitting room. Wonderful breakfast included. Moderate.

Wycombe Inn 1031 Millcreek Road, Wycombe (ZIP 18980) 215-598-7000 This is a historic hotel that has been remodeled with lovely, quite modern suites, most of them with fireplaces and small kitchens. There is a romantic restaurant and bar. Moderate.

Stockton Inn 1 Main Street, P.O. Box C, Stockton, NJ (ZIP 08559) 609-397-1250 Technically not in Bucks County, but this is right across the river from New

Hope—and what could be more Bucks County than that? This is a pretty place with lovely rooms, some with canopy beds, and suites. A romantic atmosphere pervades this whole district. Inexpensive to moderate.

Phoenix

Maricopa Manor 15 West Pasadena Avenue (ZIP 85013) 800-292-6403 or 602-274-6302; fax: 602-266-3904 This hotel has an enticing Spanish Mission–style architecture: stucco, arched doorways, and red tile. The place is on the formal and fancy side—lovely beds (some four-posters), fluffy feather beds, and fireplaces. There is a heated pool and hot tub. Lots of privacy—including a second building that has three suites. Mornings begin with a breakfast basket delivered to each door. Inexpensive to expensive.

Arizona Biltmore Twenty-fourth Street and Missouri Avenue (ZIP 85016) 800-950-0086 Staying at this place is an experience. It is a masterpiece of architecture and is a mixture of desert and Mayan atmosphere. The great public spaces overshadow the rooms, but the grounds and general luxurious service of the place make up for it. Expensive, except in the summer.

The Boulders 34631 North Tom Darlington Drive, Carefree (ZIP 85377) 800-553-1717 Want perfect privacy for your romantic weekend? We recommend this very pricey, very wonderful retreat. They are all private casetas, with southwestern style. Beautiful big bathrooms (though some have only showers!) and a lovely sitting area. All the amenities (including wonderful salsa and chips) and great pools, golf course, spa, and restaurants. Very expensive, but there are times of the year when you can get a good deal here.

. . . . *In Sedona*

L'Auberge   301 L'Auberge Lane, P.O. Box B (ZIP 86339) 800-272-6777 Secluded cottages, fireplaces, wrought-iron beds, some with canopies. Refrigerators in rooms. Moderate to expensive.

Enchantment   525 Boynton Canyon Road (ZIP 86336) 800-826-4180 Nestled in an exceptionally stunning canyon. Chic casetas, a perfect place for a getaway. Feel like one of the rich and famous. Tennis, swimming, hiking, riding, and romance. Excellent food. Expensive.

Portland

Governor Hotel   611 Southwest Tenth Street (ZIP 97205) 503-224-3400 or 800-554-3456 This hotel's turn-of-the-century atmosphere sets the scene. The deluxe rooms feature sitting areas, high ceilings (some with skylights), and Jacuzzis. Some of the suites have fireplaces. It's definitely romantic. Expensive.

Hotel Vintage Plaza   422 Southwest Broadway (ZIP 97205) 503-228-1212 or 800-243-0555 This is one of those wonderful lobbies that set the mood. There are dark paneled walls, beautiful bouquets of fresh flowers, and an operating fireplace. Book one of the nine Starlight Rooms, which have beautiful views from very large picture windows. Luxurious linens and all the amenities. If you really want to splurge, there are townhouse units with full kitchens, soaking tubs, living rooms, and loft bedrooms. Expensive.

. . . . *Near Portland*

THE COAST

Stephanie Inn   2740 South Pacific, Cannon Beach (ZIP 97110)   800-633-3466   or   503-436-2221   We couldn't resist this one. It is perfect—right on Cannon Beach, a wide, stunning, often windy expanse that is punctuated by wonderful rock formations. Most, but not all, rooms look out on the water. Each is romantically decorated, and the public rooms are very inviting. You can also stroll into town, which is absolutely charming—though much better if you avoid the crowded summer season. All the amenities: fireplaces, Jacuzzi tubs, and some rooms with little decks or balconies. And guess what—no small children allowed. Moderate.

Channel House   35 Ellingson Street, Depoe Bay (ZIP 97341)   800-447-2140   This blue frame building sets you right over the crashing surf; it is an astoundingly romantic setting. Make sure you get one with a great view and its own deck. Some also have very private hot tubs. Inexpensive to expensive

San Diego

The U.S. Grant Hotel   326 Broadway (ZIP 92101) 619-232-3121   This landmark 1886 hotel has been totally redone and now has some of its old grand manner back. It is right in the heart of downtown and close to Horton Plaza and the restaurant and theater quarter. Go higher up and get a water view. Inexpensive to moderate.

The Hotel Del Coronado   1500 Orange (ZIP 92118)   800-HOTEL DEL or 619-435-6611   A true landmark on the National Historic Register. It is wonderful from the outside and right on the beach—but inside it is too often utilized by conventions. Still, the location is intensely romantic. See if you can get a larger room with a great view. Moderate to expensive.

Horton Grand Hotel   311 Island Avenue (ZIP 92101)   800-542-1886 or 619-544-1886   Located in the Gaslamp Quarter, where the restaurants, clubs, and theaters liven up the streets. All the suites have fireplaces. Ask about romantic packages. Moderate to expensive.

. . . . Near San Diego

LA JOLLA
La Valencia   1132 Prospect Street (ZIP 92037) 800-451-0772 or 619-454-0771; fax: 619-456-3921 This is just what you would hope a getaway hotel would be: small, charming, private, cozy, and with a view of the

ocean. Your room might be small, but as long it has that ocean view, you won't mind. This is such a pretty hotel. Moderate to expensive.

RANCHO SANTE FE

Inn at Rancho Sante Fe   5951 Linea del Cielo (ZIP 92067)   800-843-4661 or 858-756-1131   This is an incredibly lovely and prosperous suburb of San Diego with an elegant, casual feel. Most of the rooms have fireplaces and/or patios. There are tennis courts, a pool, six hot tubs, and some very inviting old California public rooms and restaurant. Moderate to expensive.

San Francisco

The Archbishops Mansion   1000 Fulton Street (ZIP 94117)   415-563-7872   An amazing place to stay. There are elegant appointments, and just grand public rooms. The majority of rooms have fireplaces, and quite a few are suites with their own sitting rooms. Each room is named, and you can write for the brochure and see them before you choose. You will find this place baronial, including the service and hospitality. Mention our book. Inexpensive to expensive.

The Sherman House   2160 Green Street (ZIP 94123)   415-563-3600; fax: 415-563-1882   This is a small but elegant hotel. Rooms all have canopy beds, feather duvets, and marble fireplaces. It feels very much like old San Francisco here. You are located in the Pacific Heights area, close to great walking and shopping on

Union Street. Some rooms have spectacular views. Expensive.

The Huntington on Nob Hill   1075 California Street (ZIP 94108)   415-474-5400; fax: 415-474-6227 This is the place to feel like an elegant San Francisco couple having a discreet affair while on a business mission. The hotel has a clubby, exclusive feel—especially by the romantic fireplace bar. There is fine service, even a free limo to the business district. Moderate to expensive.

Hotel Monaco   501 Geary Road (ZIP 94102) 415-292-0100   This hotel (also located in Seattle) is ideal for a romantic getaway. You get the kind of style— bright colors, high concept furniture and great details that you only get in the classiest places. The San Francisco hotel features an "Oh Baby, Baby" weekend, which includes one of their Mediterranean Suites, two 30-minute massages given either in your suite or in the hotel's spa, in-room martinis, wine, morning newspapers and continental breakfast. Expensive.

. . . . *Near San Francisco*

WOODSIDE
The Lodge at Skylonda   16350 Skyline Boulevard (ZIP 94062)   800-851-2222; fax: 415-788-0150   This log-and-stone lodge combines fitness with romance.

Rooms have decks and soaking tubs, and there are endless hiking trails to try out. This is a full-fledged spa that offers classes on New Age topics. A wonderful, healthy kitchen. Expensive.

THE COAST

Seal Cove Inn   221 Cypress, Moss Beach (ZIP 94038)   650-728-7325   or   800-995-9987   for reservations.   A small country inn, with plenty of walking trails down to the beach or along the top for scenic vistas. Every room is a winner—with fireplaces and views of the gorgeous coastal water and cliffs. One of the most romantic landscapes in this world. Best of all, not expensive. Moderate.

Pelican Inn   10 Pacific Way, Muir Beach (ZIP 94965)   415-383-6000   The inn has a decidedly dressy English turn. Each room is very romantic; they all have canopy beds and lavish appointments. Moderate to expensive.

MONTEREY

Spindrift Inn   652 Cannery Row (ZIP 93940) 800-841-1879 or 831-646-8900   You have a lovely view on the inn's own beach, and inside you can feel snug in the always surprising Monterey weather. There are wood-burning fireplaces and big fluffy down comforters. There is also a wonderful wharf to walk—and that terrific aquarium, which is kind of romantic, too, if it isn't crowded. Moderate.

PACIFIC GROVE
The Martine Inn   255 Oceanview Boulevard (ZIP
93950)   800-852-5588 or 831-373-3388   This is a wonderful getaway—less chic than Carmel and Monterey, but
still lovely and much more reasonable than its more famous neighboring towns. The inn has wonderful Victorian rooms and nice suites with magnificent beds. There
is a romantic view of the ocean from the breakfast room.
Inexpensive to expensive.

CARMEL
The Highlands Inn   Highway One P.O. Box 1700
(ZIP 93921)   831-624-3801   This is a romantic place
and a romantic hotel. Walking Carmel's shops and
beaches is romantic—no matter what the weather. Many
of the suites here have fireplaces and kitchens, and
they are a good value out of season. Not all the bedrooms
have great views, but most of the public rooms do. Expensive.

. . . . *The Napa Valley*
   Many wonderful getaways here, among them:

CALISTOGA
Foothill House   3037 Foothill Boulevard (ZIP
94515)   800-942-6933   A lovely farmhouse with good
food served and fine wine tasting in the afternoons (what a
wonderful break that would be!). Lovers should ask for the
private cottage. Regular rooms vary. We like the ones with

four-poster beds and Jacuzzis. Evening cookies, sherry, or champagne. Mention our book. Moderate to expensive.

Cottage Grove Inn   1711 Lincoln Avenue (ZIP 94515)   800-799-2284 or 707-942-8400; fax: 707-942-2653   These are simply wonderful cottages, each with a wicker rocking chair on its front porch, a fireplace, superior sound systems and VCRs, and soaking tubs. Too romantic for words. Moderate.

St. Helena
Inn at Southbridge   1020 Main Street (ZIP 94574) 707-967-9400 or 800-520-6800   New and lovely, right in the charming town of St. Helena. Has access to a very fancy spa at Meadowood, and another spa will be opening across the road. King-size beds, wood-burning fireplaces and tastefully decorated low-key rooms. Very good Italian restaurant on premises. Wine tasting, horseback riding. Moderate to expensive

The Zinfandel Inn   800 Zinfandel Lane (ZIP 94574)   707-963-3512   Since this area has some things in common with Provence, in the south of France, French themes predominate here. This is a chateau-like retreat, and each room has a spa tub, fireplace, and balcony. Inexpensive to expensive.

Yountville
The Crossroads Inn   6380 Silverado Trail (ZIP 94599)   707-944-0855   This inn has only four rooms, but each is very romantic. The rooms are done up in a

charming French provincial theme. You can have your breakfast delivered to your room, sip a glass of wine at night, and enjoy pastoral views from the deck. Moderate.

. . . . *Sonoma*

Sonoma Mission Inn and Spa 18140 Highway 12, Boyes Hot Springs (ZIP 95476) 800-862-4945 or 707-938-9000; fax: 707-996-5358 This quintessential resort is known for its world-class spa, superb dining, and award-winning service. Surrounded by eight acres of eucalyptus-shaded grounds. The perfect romantic getaway located in the heart of wine country. Ask about special romance packages. Expensive.

GLEN ELLEN
Beltane Ranch 11775 Sonoma Highway (ZIP 95442) 707-996-6501 This is a small inn on a big piece of property—1600 acres, to be exact. There are five very nice rooms and a great double-decker porch that has a swing and hammocks. Talk about relaxation and privacy. Your extremely nice price also includes breakfast. Moderate.

LITTLE RIVER
Heritage House 5200 North Highway One, Little River (ZIP 95456) 800-235-5885 or 707-937-5885 This is kind of cheating, since the hotel is a good three and a half hours from San Francisco. But if you're really looking for romance—well, what can we say but that this was the place they shot the movie *Same Time Next Year*. Nestled against the hillside overlooking the coastline, it

feels like you are in both California and France. Mention our book. Moderate, since the price includes breakfast and dinner.

Seattle

Hotel Monaco   110 4th Avenue (ZIP 98101)   206-621-1770; fax: 206-621-7799   The hotel (also located in San Francisco) is ideal for a romantic getaway. You get the kind of style—bright colors, high concept furniture—that you usually get in the classiest places. The Seattle hotel features an "Oh Baby, Baby" weekend, which includes one of their Mediterranean Suites, champagne and truffles at bedside, a Jacuzzi thoughtfully accompanied by Aveda bath salts and a keepsake CD with just the right mood music. Add the included room service breakfast and you have a perfect getaway. Expensive.

Olympic Four Seasons   411 University Street (ZIP 98101)   800-223-8772 or 206-621-1700   This is one of the elegant, great, old hotels, completely updated and well-run. There is a very nice health club and pool, and most rooms are nice. For a little more space, ask for a junior suite. The restaurants are romantic, and you are in a great location to walk downtown or to the waterfront. Ask about their special romantic weekends. Expensive.

The Inn at the Market   86 Pine Street (ZIP 98101) 800-446-4484 or 206-443-3600   This is a European-style hotel with a small flower-filled lobby, a great restaurant across the way, and a farmer's market at your fingertips.

Some of the suites are wonderful—and reasonable, for two floors, views of the sound and city, and French flowered rooms that are cheerful and comfortable. All rooms have access to the perfect rooftop garden that looks over Puget Sound and shipping lanes. Moderate.

The Alexis   1007 First Avenue (ZIP 98104)   206-624-4844 or 800-426-7033; fax: 206-621-9009   This is a very tasteful hotel, with superb service. Some rooms have fireplaces. It is near the Pike Place Market and Pioneer Square. Small and service-oriented, they will cater to your every need. The rooms are decorated in Northwest subtle shades with flattering mellow colors. Very good restaurants. Expensive.

The Edgewater Hotel   2411 Alaskan Way, Pier 67 (ZIP 98121)   206-728-7000 or 800-624-0670   This is Seattle's only waterfront hotel. It has a wonderful lodge feel, all done with light pine so that the effect is light rather than dark. The theme carries through to the rooms—by all means insist on one on the water side. Great views in the lounge and restaurant as well. Moderate.

. . . . *Near Seattle*

SNOQUALMIE
Salish Lodge   6501 Railroad Avenue (ZIP 98065), about one half hour from Seattle   800-826-6124   A personal favorite. This sort of Ralph Lauren–decorated lodge

sits above the thundering 260-feet cliffs of Snoqualmie Falls. The rooms are luxurious and spacious: Each has down comforters, a hot tub, and a fireplace. The dining room itself has private rooms over the falls that are terribly romantic; sweethearts are discreetly left alone. A good health club and a wonderful area for hiking, biking, and fishing in the shadow of Mount Si. Reasonable midweek; expensive on the weekends.

WHIDBEY ISLAND

The Inn at Langley   400 First Street, Langley (ZIP 98260)   360-221-3033   Another favorite. This international-style small hotel has all 24 rooms facing the water and Saratoga Passage. Each room has a hot tub with an unobstructed view and a fireplace. The rooms, like the hotel, have a Northwest-Japanese peaceful feel— you may never want to leave bed, even though the town and the island have great restaurants and are worth exploring. Moderate to expensive.

Guest House Bed-and-Breakfast Cottages— Greenbank   24371 State Route 525 (ZIP 98253)   360-678-3115   This group of cottages are keyed to a honeymoon atmosphere. They are lovely log cottages with pine paneling, skylights, private soaking tubs, VCRs and TVs, kitchens, fireplaces, and big beds with down comforters. The kitchens are stocked with everything you need for breakfast the next morning. If this isn't enough for you, there is a larger log house for rent that is really spectacular. Everyone has access to an outdoor pool and hot tub. Moderate.

THE SAN JUAN ISLANDS

Inn at Swift's Bay   856 Port Stanley Road, Lopez Island (ZIP 98261)   360-468-3636   The inn itself is lovely—although intensely decorated near, not at, the beach, and perhaps too close quarters for our lovers. What you want here is their private cottage—separate from the inn—but you can go there for wonderful breakfasts and other parts of the island for wonderful lunches and dinners. The separate cottage is truly romantic—a view that gives you your own ocean, and a place to create the world's most romantic weekend. Total privacy. Moderate to expensive.

Tucson

Arizona Inn   2200 East Elm Street (ZIP 85719) 520-325-1541   This is a private, quiet getaway. There are lovely grounds and fountains, an inviting pool, and the inclination to pay attention only to each other. There is a great lounge. Moderate.

Westward Look Resort   245 East Ina Road (ZIP 85704)   520-297-1151   This is a laid-back resort with three pools, three spas, a fitness center, and a walking and nature trail. The rooms are large and have either views of the city or mountains, beamed ceilings, and wet bars with a sitting area. There is a quiet charm to the clustered southwestern buildings. You could be focused on each other here. Moderate.

Lodge on the Desert   306 North Alvernon Way (ZIP 85711)   800-456-5634   This has a hacienda theme, and the best places to stay are the adobe-style casetas with their welcoming verandas. The rooms are spacious, and many have wood-burning fireplaces. The place has a lot of charm. Inexpensive to moderate.

Washington, D.C.

The Morrison-Clark Inn   1015 11th Street NW (ZIP 20001)   202-898-1200   This hotel is located in the middle of Washington and has been placed on the national List of Historic Places. There is a modern addition, and rooms vary from small to luxurious; ones on the outside facing the street are larger, with balconies. Ones on the inner courtyard are smaller, but quieter. Ask for a room with atmosphere: some have antiques and beds with canopies. Inexpensive rooms and moderate suites.

The Willard Continental   1401 Pennsylvania Avenue NW (ZIP 20004) 202-628-9100; fax: 202-637-7326 A hotel with a past. The lobby isn't too impressive, but you do feel as if you are experiencing some piece of our country's history. There are some nice bars to hang out in. Most rooms are a good size and tastefully decorated. Moderate to expensive.

The Jefferson 1200 16th and M Streets NW (ZIP 20036) 202-347-2200; fax: 202-331-7982 This is the hotel that will show you how visiting politicians (and politicians having affairs) live when they stay in a Washington hotel. This is restrained elegance. All the rooms have antiques or reproductions, and the bathrooms are large and lovely, as are the rooms. There is access to a health club and swimming pool. Rooms have CD players and VCRs—and everything else you need to feel like the Power People. Expensive.

Near Washington, D.C.

. . . . Virginia

FAIRFAX

The Baliwick Inn 4023 Chain Bridge Road (ZIP 22030) 703-691-2266 or 800-366-7666; fax: 703-934-2112 Just a beautiful place, with some of the most handsome bedrooms you've ever seen. A fabulous food place, but the rooms are worth a visit on their own. There are impressive four-posters, hung with exquisite fabrics. Some of the rooms have Jacuzzis; all have lovely towels, linens and amenities. This is a place that has many rooms perfect for lovers. Inexpensive to moderate.

FLINT HILL

Caledonia Farm 47 Dearing Road, Flint Hill (ZIP 22627) 800-262-1812 or 540-675-3693 Just a little over an hour away from Washington, but light-years away emotionally. This nineteenth-century stone manor house is a historic landmark and is still a working cattle farm. There are lovely bedrooms with fireplaces and antiques, and amazing views of the Blue Ridge Mountains. There is also a very fine kitchen. Go for the one suite; otherwise, you might not get your own bathroom. This is a bit more rustic than most of the places we've mentioned, but it has romance written all over it. Inexpensive for the rooms, moderate for the suite.

Four and Twenty Blackbirds 650 Zachary Taylor Highway (ZIP 22627) 540-675-1111 Close to the Inn at Little Washington but a whole lot less expensive, so you could stay here and make one splurge dinner reservation over there. Each room is beautifully decorated and romantic, with marble baths and fireplaces. Moderate to expensive.

Middleburg
Red Fox Inn 2 East Washington Street (ZIP 20117) 800-223-1728 or 540-687-6301; fax: 540-687-6053 This place absolutely reeks of hunt country ambience. Middleburg is a classy place, and staying here makes you feel as if you belong. The rooms aren't large, but they are charming. There is a wonderful tavern, a good restaurant, and some of the loveliest American countryside anywhere to explore for antiques or history. Moderate (and includes breakfast).

Williamsburg
Liberty Rose Bed-and-Breakfast 1022 Jamestown Road (ZIP 23185) 800-545-1825 This establishment

was made for romance: There are queen-size four-posters, fluffy duvets, claw-footed tubs, marble showers, and period fabrics. There are also all those gadgets—like VCRs—that we need for this weekend. Inexpensive for a room; moderate for one of the three suites.

WASHINGTON
The Inn at Little Washington   Middle and Main Streets (ZIP 22747)   540-675-3800   This is rated as the best hotel in the South by many. People who are serious about food rave about the restaurant, and reservations are hard to come by. The twelve bedrooms are beautifully put together, with wonderful chintz patterns and comfortable furniture. There are VCRs and other amenities in the rooms. People come here to be treated well, and they are. Expensive.

WHITE POST
L'Auberge Provençal   13630 Lord Fairfax Highway, Boyze (ZIP 26620)   800-638-1702   This is a place with the personal touch. The owners will tell you how to see everything in the area, and they are also intimately involved in the day-to day-running of the place, including the kitchen. The food is wonderful and the rooms are all different, all charming. Ask about them: Some have canopy beds and fireplaces, or they might face the garden. Moderate.

. . . . *Maryland*

ANNAPOLIS
The Maryland Inn   16 Main Street (ZIP 21401)
800-847-8882   This is a wonderfully shaped building in
the center of town. The town is close to D.C. and worth
walking around in. The colonial rooms are each unique,
full of antiques, and very comfortable. Good service and
amenities. Moderate.

MIDDLETOWN
Stone Manor   5820 Carroll Boyer Road (ZIP
21769)   301-473-5454   Beautiful house on a lovely
piece of property. Views of fields, woods, and ponds. Originally built in the eighteenth century, it has had several ad-
ditions and renovations. Very elegant and very much
organized around food—definitely for serious gourmets.
Still, the rooms are also wonderful. There are five suites
with queen-size four-poster and other romantic beds.
They also have Jacuzzi tubs (sometimes for two) and vary
with other nice touches, such as sitting rooms, a special
shower that hits you with six jets, and a tub with underwa-
ter lighting. Moderate to expensive (includes breakfast).

OXFORD
Robert Morris Inn   314 North Morris Street (ZIP
21654)   410-226-5111; fax: 410-226-5744   There are
several kinds of accommodations grouped as the inn, including a lodge and cottages. One of them is the Robert

Morris Lodge on the Tred Avon River, and a room there with a view of the river would be just right. The rooms have a country motif, with claw-footed tubs in some of them. Some rooms are more updated than others. The inn can send you a brochure to help you choose which room would suit you. Moderate.

CANADA

Montreal

Ritz-Carlton Kempinski   1228 Sherbrook Street West (Postal Code H3G 1H6)   800-363-0366 or 514-842-4212; fax: 514-842-2268   We hate to nominate the obvious, but this is such a lovely hotel, we had to. Edwardian elegance; rooms are very pretty and many have fireplaces. The Ritz Garden is a very romantic place to have lunch during good weather. Health club privileges. Expensive.

Auberge Hatley   325 Chemin Virgin CP 330 North Hatley (Postal Code J0B 2C0)   819-842-2451; fax: 819-842-2907   A member of the prestigious and almost always wonderful group of Relais and Chateau. On a lake, not too far a drive away. Beautiful sleigh and canopy beds, with wonderful activities for every season. Gourmet food. Expensive.

Quebec

Hôtel l'Eau à la Bouche   3003 Boulevard Sainte-Adèle, Sainte-Adèle, Quebec (Postal Code J8B 2N6) 514-229-2991; fax: 514-229-7573   A member of the Relais and Chateau, it is an easy drive from Montreal. Wonderful French ambience; romantic rooms with fireplaces and terraces. Excellent dining. Moderate to expensive.

Toronto

Park Plaza Hotel   4 Avenue Road (Postal Code M5R 2E8)   800-977-4197 or 416-924-5471; fax: 416-924-4933   Old World charm and one of the great romantic rooftop restaurants, with beautiful views of the city. Indoor pool and fitness center, with interesting neighborhood shops to look at during your break. Moderate to expensive.

Elora Inn   77 Millstreet, Elora, Ontario (Postal Code N0B 1S0)   519-846-5356; fax: 519-846-9180   Astoundingly romantic 150-year-old mill inn placed over the dramatic falls of the Grand River. Antiques, quilts, fireside dining overlooking the falls. Rooms have vaulted ceilings, stone walls, fireplaces, and four-poster or brass beds. An hour's drive from Toronto. Moderate.

Millcroft Inn   55 John Street, Alton, Ontario (Postal Code L0N 1A0)   519-941-8111; fax: 519-941-

9192   Another find. Forty minutes from Toronto. Wonderful two-story cabins with fireplaces—outdoor hot tubs in some—and private decks. In a most beautiful setting—100 acres of woodland. Serious restaurant. Moderate.

Vancouver

Wedgewood Hotel   845 Homby Street (Postal Code V6Z 1V1)   604-689-7777 or 800-663-0666   The Four Seasons may have better views (and is also a good choice in this city), but it's hard to beat this hotel for intimate European elegance. This feels like a private, personal hotel, and many of the rooms feel like small apartments because they have sitting rooms and fireplaces. Decks, too. Moderate to expensive.

Laburnum Cottage   1388 Terrace Avenue, North Vancouver (Postal Code V7R 1B4)   604-988-4877 About a half an hour from Vancouver, four rooms in the main house (with baths), and five cottages—all of which are absolutely charming. One cottage has a kitchen, fireplace, and skylights. Down comforters and all the right details, including gourmet breakfast delivered to your doorstep in the morning. Discount to our readers. Expensive to moderate.

RiverRun Cottages   4551 River Road West, Ladner (Postal Code V4K 1R9)   604-946-7778; fax: 604-940-1970   Completely charming cottages and floating houseboats. Some with lofts, soaking tubs, kitchens, fireplaces, and water views. All have refrigerators and microwaves.

Great respect for privacy. Breakfast delivered to your door. Special romance packages; mention our book. Moderate.

THE GULF ISLANDS

Hastings House on Salt Spring Island, British Columbia   160 Upper Ganges Road (Postal Code V8K 2S2)   800-661-9255 or 250-537-2362   This place is just too perfect. There are very different kinds of wonderful accommodations, from rooms at the main house to duplex separate buildings. All come with their own down comforters and terry-cloth robes. Some have wood-burning fireplaces and kitchenettes. Most have stunning views of the sound. The main house is a wonderful English residence that is used as the dining room and for tea and sherry time. The food is splendid and people are left alone—or spoken to—as much as they want. Most of the herbs and vegetables are grown on site. Expensive.

Victoria

Abigail's   906 McClure Street (Postal Code V8V 3E7)   250-388-5363   This rather large bed-and-breakfast bends over backward to be romantic. Fireplaces, comforters, and antique furnishings and appointments. Very pretty throughout, but each room is quite different, so ask. Moderate to expensive.

Laurel Point Inn   680 Montreal Street (Postal Code V8V 1Z8)   250-386-8721 or   800-663-7667   Modern and large, but don't let that fool you. The suites are affordable and fabulous, with drop-dead views of Victrial Harbour. Pitched beamed roofs, marble baths, spas in the room—floor-to-ceiling windows to take it all in. Expensive.

Prior House   620 St. Charles Street (Postal Code V8S 3N7)   250-592-8847   Lavish. Huge Victorian mansion on gorgeous grounds. Many of the rooms match the fabulous downstairs—some with fireplaces, French doors that open to a private patio, and spa tubs. There is high tea, and breakfast can be delivered to your room. You will feel as if you are in a movie. Moderate to expensive.

APPENDIX 3

Mail-Order Catalogs

THE FOUR FOLLOWING MAIL-ORDER CATALOGS for sex toys, books, and adult videos were all selected because they guarantee to be discreet and protect your privacy. Items and packages are sent in plain wrappers. All four promise to never sell, rent, or trade your name to another business or organization. We also like these catalogs because they contain tasteful drawings of the merchandise.

Eve's Garden

PHONE: 800-848-3837 or 212-757-8651
FAX: 617-227-5342
E-MAIL: huntress@evesgarden.com
WEB SITE: http://www.evesgarden.com

STORE LOCATION: 119 West 57th Street, Suite 1201, New
York, NY 10019

*Orders taken by phone from 11 A.M. to 7 P.M., Monday
through Saturday, Eastern Standard Time, or twenty-four hours
via the Web site. Catalog costs $4.00, which can be applied to your
first purchase.*

*Discreetly located on the twelfth floor of an office building in
the heart of New York, a couple of blocks from the Plaza, this surprising sex shop provides a comfortable setting and first-rate advice
about the merchandise, including spanking accessories, dildos, and
vibrating panties that are remote controlled by your honey.*

Good Vibrations

PHONE: 800-289-8423 or 415-974-8980
FAX: 415-974-8989
MAIL: 938 Howard Street, Suite 101, San Francisco,
CA 94103
STORE LOCATIONS: 1210 Valencia Street, San Francisco,
CA 94110
2504 San Pablo Avenue, Berkeley, CA
94702
E-MAIL: goodvibe@well.com
WEB SITE: http://www.goodvibes.com

*Orders taken by phone Monday through Saturday from 7 A.M.
to 7 P.M. Pacific Standard Time.*

*In addition to the free Good Vibrations toy catalog, you can
request the free Sexuality Library catalog of books and videos. Together, these catalogs offer a first-rate selection of everything you
need for a memorable weekend.*

Indulgenz

PHONE: 888-4-INDULGE (446-3854)
FAX: 818-883-3444
MAIL: EBP, Inc., 19528 Ventura Blvd., #579,
            Tarzana, CA 91356
E-MAIL: indulgenz@aol.com
WEB SITE: http://www.indulgenz.com

Orders taken twenty-four hours a day. This hip, upscale catalog was designed for couples who believe that energizing their relationship is of utmost importance. In addition to selective sex toys, adult videos and books, this catalog features sexy lingerie, casual and evening wear. Fabulous bath products and aromatic candles and incense make this practically a one-stop shop for a romantic weekend retreat. In fact, they feature a variety of kits ready to toss in your luggage.

Xandria

PHONE: 800-242-2823
FAX: 415-468-3912
MAIL: 165 Valley Drive, San Francisco, CA 94131
WEB SITE: http://www.xandria.com

Orders taken twenty-four hours on Monday through Friday, and until 4:30 P.M. Pacific Standard Time on Saturday.

Xandria's catalog costs $4.00, which can be applied to your first purchase. Xandria's Web site is a very popular place to get erotic playthings; sign up there for their interesting and informative electronic newsletter.

FOR OTHER RECOMMENDED PERSONAL ITEMS

Alaris of Sonoma

PHONE: 707-939-7566
FAX: 707-939-7567
MAIL: 19229 Sonoma Highway, Sonoma, CA 95476

   Romantic and sensual all-natural handmade soaps, bath oils and other bath products.

Condomania

PHONE: 800-9CONDOM (926-6366) or 323-930-5330
WEB SITE: http://www.condomania.com
STORE LOCATIONS: 351 Bleecker Street, New York, NY 10014
               7306 Melrose, Los Angeles, CA 90046

   Orders taken by phone Monday through Saturday from 9 A.M. to 6 P.M. Pacific Standard Time.

   America's first condom store is now one of the Internet's premier safer sex sites, featuring over three hundred types of condoms, lubricants, and other romance products and gift items. Visit the Condom Wizard, an interactive search guide, to help you find the perfect condom for your tastes and needs.

Condom Sense

PHONE: 888-776-2906
WEB SITE: http://www.condoms.net

   Orders taken by phone Monday through Saturday from 9 A.M. to 6 P.M. Pacific Standard Time.

Another great Web site for good deals on variety packs of condoms and lubricants so you can experiment to find your favorites. Buying condoms in large quantities is economical and keeps you prepared for fun in bed.

Frederick's of Hollywood

PHONE: 800-323-9525 or 310-637-7770
FAX: 323-467-5803
WEB SITE: http://www.fredericks.com

Orders taken by phone twenty-four hours a day. Catalog is free. Or call to find the closest retail store among the several hundred in the nationwide chain. Lacier, racier lingerie will fit some people's fantasies more than Victoria's Secret designs. It's all a matter of personal taste.

Lubricants (Where to go for our favorites)

☆ *Astroglide* is sold in most catalogs listed in this book and is available in some drugstores, too. For a free sample, you can call 800-848-5900.

☆ *Bonne Forme* is a unique lubricant that simulates natural feminine secretions. Designed by the nationally renowned gynecologist Penny Wise Budoff, M.D., this glycerin-based lube with aloe vera can be ordered at 800-426-0034.

☆ *ID Millennium* is a velvety-smooth silicone-based formula that makes it much longer-lasting and slicker than water-based lubricants—super concentrated, just a tiny drop works wonders. (Besides, any more might stain your sheets.) Silicon lubricants won't harm latex condoms, are tasteless, odorless, and hypoallergenic. Sold in specialty stores and catalogs or through the manufacturer, Westridge Laboratories in Irvine, CA; call 800-646-2096 or visit its Web site: http://www.idlube@aol.com.

☆   *ID Juicy Lube* (another Westridge product; see above for order information) is for those who prefer a water-based formula, and it comes in a variety of tropical flavors like passion fruit, pina colada, strawberry kiwi, and succulent watermelon for those who want to fantasize that they're on an island vacation. Non-staining formula contains no sugar or dyes.

Tender Loving Things, Inc.

PHONE: 800-486-2896
E-MAIL: info@tenderlovingthings.com
WEB SITE: http://www.tenderlovingthings.com

The creator of the Happy Massager®, TLT sells its products in five thousand retail outlets throughout the United States and Canada. In addition to the two sizes of massagers, TLT sells wonderful massage oils, body lotions, bubble bath, bath salts, and aromatherapy soaps. Call to get their catalog with more products for relaxation and romance or to locate the store nearest you that carries their products.

Tom and Sally's

PHONE: 800-827-0800 or 802-254-4200
E-MAIL: tomsally@together.net
WEB SITE: http://www.tomandsallys.com

Makers of the homemade "Chocolate Body Paint" (great on ice cream, too) and "Chocolate Body Powder" (makes rich cocoa and comes with a purple ostrich feather). Expensive, but worth it.

Victoria's Secret Catalog
PHONE: 800-888-8200
MAIL: P.O. Box 16589, Columbus, OH 43216

Offers an extensive collection of sleepwear and undergarments for both women and men, tastefully and sensually displayed on live models. Orders taken twenty-four hours every day, and filled in seven to ten working days. Victoria's Secret operates a nationwide chain of retail stores; call the toll-free number if you need help locating the store nearest you.

Happy Massager® Guide

To buy a Happy Massager®, see Tender
Loving Things in "Mail-Order Catalogs"

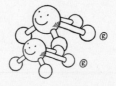

Massage Is Caring Touch

Caring touch is when the hands become an extension of
the heart. For thousands of years, massage has been one
of the principal means of focusing caring touch to relieve
the body naturally of unhealthy tension and pain.

This guide is intended to introduce you to using the
Happy Massager®, a massage tool invented for you to
help make massage easy and fun. Try some of the tips we
put in this guide and you'll find out why we say, "It's hard
to believe that something so simple can feel so good!"

𝒯HE 𝓑ASICS

✧ Start at the base of the back and move upward with slow, even strokes.

✧ Massage toward the heart!

✧ Vary pressure depending on the sensitivity of your body. Muscular areas may take more pressure. Be sure to stop if painful.

✧ Use caution when massaging pregnant women, as their bodies are sensitive.

✧ Don't massage directly on the spine or other bony areas.

✧ Experiment and **have fun!**

The **Large Happy Massager®** works best for large hands and large muscle groups such as the legs, back, chest, and shoulders.

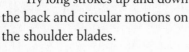

Try long strokes up and down the back and circular motions on the shoulder blades.

The Happy Massager® fits perfectly on the base of the skull.

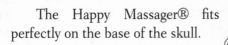

Try light pressure on the head. Massage your head to help release tension in your entire body!

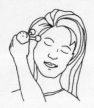

Circle the temples with care. It feels good!

Massage the stomach carefully with gentle circles!

MERIDIANS AND ACUPRESSURE POINTS

The unique design of the Happy Massager® stimulates meridians and acupressure points. The lines below show where meridians are, and the hearts represent acupressure points. Meridians are channels of energy that run throughout your entire body. They can be compared to a highway. When there is a buildup of excess energy (such as stress, or a knot in your muscle) a traffic jam is created. Massage can break up traffic jams and reopen blocked passageways by helping release tension! Acupressure points are found along meridians. Each point corresponds to specific areas in your body. By focusing pressure on different points, you can bring attention and energy to those parts of your body.

To learn more about how to apply acupressure points to cultivate intimacy and intensify sexual pleasure, you can order instructional videos from the *Acupressure for Lovers* Series. We like the one titled "Preparing for Love: Acupressure Massage for Foreplay and Lovemaking." To order, call the Acupressure Institute in Berkeley, California, at 800-442-2232 or 510-845-1059.

APPENDIX 5

Recommended Adult Videos

WE USED FOUR SOURCES TO PROVIDE VIDEO
titles. The following are either highly recommended by
Good Vibrations' Sexuality Library catalog (see "Mail-Order
Catalogs") as well as *The Wise Woman's Guide to Erotic
Videos* by Angela Cohen and Sarah Garner Fox, or they are
among the top sellers from the extensive *After Midnight
Collection* (800-400-6103) or *Indulgenz* (see "Mail-Order
Catalogs") that are marked as especially appropriate for
couples' viewing.

Drama
Alexandra
Burgundy Blue
F
Hidden Obsessions
House of Dreams
Justine: Nothing to Hide 2
The Masseuse
Platinum Paradise

Comedy
Alice in Wonderland
Autobiography of a Flea
Babylon Pink
Behind the Green Door: The Sequel
Every Woman Has a Fantasy

Woman-Centered
Christine's Secret
Paris Chic
Rites of Passage
Taste of Ambrosia
Three Daughters
Trinity Brown
Urban Heat

Recommended Instructional Videos
Good Vibrations also recommends two different series of instructional videos: *Sex: A Lifelong Pleasure* and *Behind the Bedroom Door.* Volumes are sold individually or in sets.

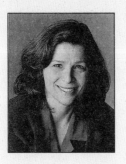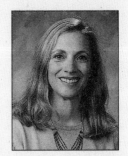

Pepper Schwartz, Ph.D., and **Janet Lever, Ph.D.**, are best known for their long tenure as columnists for *Glamour* magazine. Dr. Schwartz is a professor of sociology at the University of Washington and a recognized national authority on sexuality. She appears frequently on radio and national television, and has been featured many times on *The Oprah Winfrey Show*. The author of *American Couples: Money, Work and Sex* and other books, Dr. Schwartz hosted a sex and relationship segment on KIRO-TV in Seattle for twelve years. Dr. Lever is a professor of sociology at California State University in Los Angeles and was the senior analyst on the largest national sex survey ever tabulated. She cohosted the national cable talk show *Women on Sex* for five years, and has apppeared often in national media as an expert on sexuality.